Laboratory Manual of
Biochemistry

The Authors

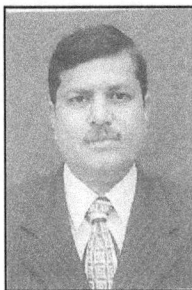

Dr. Nawaz Ahmad Khan did his B.Sc. (Ag) and M.Sc. (Ag) Biochemistry from NDUA&T, Kumarganj Faizabad in year 1988 and 1991 respectively. He got Vice Chancellor Gold Medal at M.Sc. (Biochemistry). He was awarded his Ph.D. (Biochemistry) from Gujarat Agricultural University, Junagarh in year 2000. Dr. Khan has to his credit more than 24 scientific publications and review articles which have appeared in international recognized journals. He guided M.Sc. (Ag.) Biotechnology and Ph.D. students. His research areas include Biotic Stress in Plants and Molecular Biology. He is recipient of 'Young Scientist Award' 2013 by Alumni Association of NDUA&T Kumarganj. Currently he is working as Assistant Professor, Department of Biotechnology, NDUA&T, Kumarganj, Faizabad.

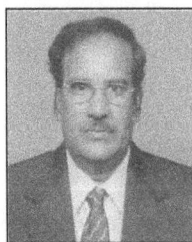

Dr. K.N. Singh did M. Phil. from JNU, New Delhi and obtained Ph.D. degree from Cambridge University, U.K. in 1990. He started his carrier as Research Associate at TERI, New Delhi and then joined Tamil Nadu Agricultural University, Coimbatore as Assistant Professor. In early 2005 he joined NDUAT as Professor in Biotechnology department. At present he is working as Head of the Departments of Biotechnology and Biochemistry. He also served as Visiting Scientist at IRRI, Philippines funded by Rockefeller Foundation. He has guided M.Sc. and Ph.D. students. Dr. Singh has published 33 research papers and review articles in journals of repute. Dr. Singh has successfully complete a number research projects funded of Govt. of India. Dr. Singh has participated delivered lectures at various National and International conferences/symposium.

Laboratory Manual of *Biochemistry*

N.A. Khan

K.N. Singh

2014

Daya Publishing House®

A Division of

Astral International Pvt. Ltd.

New Delhi – 110 002

Published by   : **Daya Publishing House®**
                            A Division of
                            Astral International Pvt. Ltd.
                            – ISO 9001:2008 Certified Company –
                            4760-61/23, Ansari Road, Darya Ganj
                            New Delhi-110 002
                            Ph. 011-43549197, 23278134
                            E-mail: info@astralint.com
                            Website: www.astralint.com

Laser Typesetting   : **Classic Computer Services**, Delhi - 110 035

Printed at   : **Replika Press Pvt. Ltd.**

PRINTED IN INDIA

Preface

The first edition of the *"Laboratory Manual of Biochemistry"* primarily designed for undergraduate and post-graduate students of Biochemistry, Horticulture and Biotechnology. Methods used with flow chart that can be understood easily. Although we have taken enough care to include operational details, it is necessary for the individual scientist and user to get conversant with the method proper.

May we request the users of this publication, scientists and scholars, to send us feedback with a view to effective improvement in subsequent editions, because it is impossible to cover all topics of biochemical analysis in one book.

We are very grateful to Vice-Chancellor of N.D. University of Agriculture & Technology, Kumarganj, Faizabad for having given us the opportunity to write the book. We would like to thanks to our Colleagues in the Department. We would like to express my thanks to Mr. Surya Mittal and Dr. B.B. Singh and staff of Astral International Pvt. Ltd. for their constant and willing help.

Kumarganj, Faizabad   **N.A. Khan**
                                                                                        K.N. Singh

Contents

1
Estimation of Titratable Acidity

Principle

Titrable acidity can be expressed conveniently in g acid per 100g or per 100ml appropriate, by using the factor appropriate to acid as follows:

1ml of 0.1N NaOH equals

Malic acid – 0.0067g

Oxalic acid – 0.0045g

Lactic acid – 0.0090g

Reagents

1. 0.1 N NaOH (4g NaOH/L.D.W.)
2. Phenolpthalein indicator 1g/100ml ethanol

Procedure

Take 5 ml juice in conical flask

↓

Volume made up to 25ml with D.W. and shake it

↓

Take 5 ml from it

↓

Add 1-2 drop of Phenolpthalein indicator

↓

Titrate it with 0.1 N NaOH till colour change to slight pink (end point)

Calculation

$$= \frac{\text{Titre} \times \text{Normality of alkali} \times \text{Volume made up} \times \text{Equivalent wt. of anhydrous citric acid} \times 100}{\text{Volume of sample taken for estimation} \times \text{Wt. or Volume of sample taken} \times 1000}$$

$$= \frac{\text{Titre} \times 0.1 \times 25 \times 64 \times 100}{5 \times 5 \times 1000} = \frac{0.33 \times 0.1 \times 25 \times 64 \times 100}{25000}$$

= 0.22 per cent

Precautions

1. Normality of NaOH should be very accurately.
2. Phenolphalein indicator should be prepared very carefully.
3. Titre value recorded very correctly when pink colour (end point) obtain.

Reference

Handbook of Analysis and Quality Control for Fruit and Vegetable Products. Second edition (1986) By-S. Ranganna, Tata Mc Graw-Hill Publishing Company Limited, New Delhi. pp. 9-10.

2

Estimation of Ascorbic Acid (Vitamin C)

Principle

Ascorbic acid reduces the 2, 6 dichlorophenol indophenol dye to a colourless leuco-base. The ascorbic acid gets oxidised to dehydroascorbic acid. Though the dye is a blue coloured compound, the end point is the appearance of pink colour. The dye is pink coloured in acid medium. Oxalic acid is used as the titrating medium.

Reagents

1. Dye Solution

    50mg of 2, 6-dichlorophenol-indophenol in

    150ml hot D.W. containing 42 mg of

    Sodium bicarbonate (Na_2HCO_3)

    ↓

    Cool it

    ↓

Dilute with 200ml distilled water (Store)

2. Metaphosphoric Acid (3 per cent)-30g/lit. (D.W.)

Standardization of Dye

Take 5ml Std. Ascorbic acid

$\downarrow$

Add 5 ml (3 per cent) metaphosphoric acid

$\downarrow$

Titrate with dye solution till slight pink

$$\text{Dye factor} = \frac{0.5}{\text{Titratable value}} \quad \text{T.V.= (4.5 to 5.5)}$$

Standardization of Ascorbic Acid

Wt. 100mg ascorbic acid

$\downarrow$

Volume made by 3 per cent metaphosphoric acid up to 100ml

$\downarrow$

1to 10 dilution with 3 per cent MPA (10ml to 100ml)

Procedure

Take 5 ml juice in conical flask

$\downarrow$

Volume made up to 25 ml with metaphosphoric acid (Homogenate)

$\downarrow$

Take 5ml aliquot

$\downarrow$

Titrate with dye solution till slight pink (end point)

Calculation

$$\text{mg of ascorbic acid content (per 100g or ml)} = \frac{\text{Titratable value} \times \text{Dye factor} \times \text{Volume made} \times 100}{\text{Aliquot taken for estimation} \times \text{Wt. or volume of sample taken for estimate}}$$

$$= \frac{(\text{T.V.}) \times 0.104 \times 25 \times 100}{5 \times 5}$$

Precautions

1. Acetic metathosphoric acid mixture may also be used instead of 4 per cent oxalic acid.

2. Dye factor should be calculated very accurately.

3. Alcohol may be used instead of acetone for extraction. The extract volume will get reduced due to evaporation at room temperature. Maintain the volume at appropriate stages. Carotenoids that are bound as esters are not estimated in this procedure.

Reference

Handbook of Analysis and Quality Control for Fruit and Vegetable Products. Second edition (1986) By-S. Ranganna, Tata Mc Graw-Hill Publishing Company Limited, New Delhi. pp. 105-106.

3

Determination of Chlorophyll

Principle

The chlorophyll are the essential components for photosynthesis and occurring chloroplasts as green pigments in all photosynthetic plant tissue. They are bound loosely to protein but are readily extracted in organic solvents. Chemically each chlorophyll molecule contains a porphyrin (tetrapyrole) nucleus with a chelated magnesium atom at the centre and a long chain hydrocarbon (Phytyl) side chain attached through a carboxylic acid group.

Chlorophyll is extracted in 80 per cent acetone and the absorption at 663nm and 645nm are read in a spectrophotometer using the absorption coefficients, the amount of chlorophyll is calculated.

Procedure

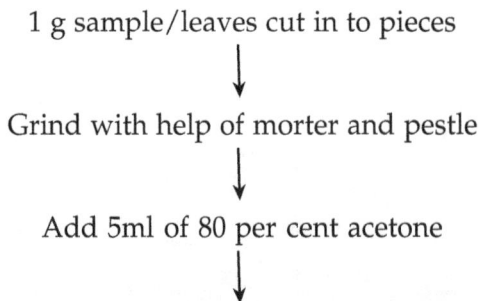

1 g sample/leaves cut in to pieces

↓

Grind with help of morter and pestle

↓

Add 5ml of 80 per cent acetone

↓

Residue grind 2-3 times by adding 80 per cent acctone

↓

Centrifuge it and final volume made up to 25ml with 80 per cent acetone

↓

Record OD at 663nm and 645nm by SP-21

Calculation

Ch. a (mg/lit) = (12.7 x OD at 663nm) – (2.69 x OD at 645nm)

Ch. b (mg/lit) = (22.9 x OD at 645nm) – (4.68 x OD at 663 nm)

Total chlorophyll (mg/lit) = (20.2xOD at 645 nm) + (8.02xOD at 663nm)

Chlorophyll

Procedure

Weight 2-10g sample (peel) = (2g peel of acid lime in 100ml diethyl ether)

↓

Add 80 per cent acetone, grind with mortar and pestle

↓

(Add calcium and magnesium carbonate in small pinch)

↓

2-3 times extraction till colourless residue

↓

Filter the extract to 100/250/500ml Volumetric flask and volume made up to mark

Purification

Take 50ml of diethyl ether in separating funnel

↓

Pipette out 25 to 50ml of Acetone extract in to this

↓

Add D.W. in to separating funnel until the water layer is apparently free of all the fat soluble pigments

$\downarrow$

Drain out the water layers

$\downarrow$

Wash the ether layer 5-10 times with 10ml protein of D.W. until the
ether layers free of acetone

$\downarrow$

Transfer the ether extract to a 100ml Vol. flask,
dilute to vol. with ether and mixed

$\downarrow$

Transfer the solution from vol. flask to amber colour reagent
bottle and add 3-5g anhydrous sodium sulphate and wait till
the solution become clear

$\downarrow$

Pipette an aliquot of this solution bottle and diluted with ether for
optimum OD read at 660 and 642.5 nm (use ether as blank)

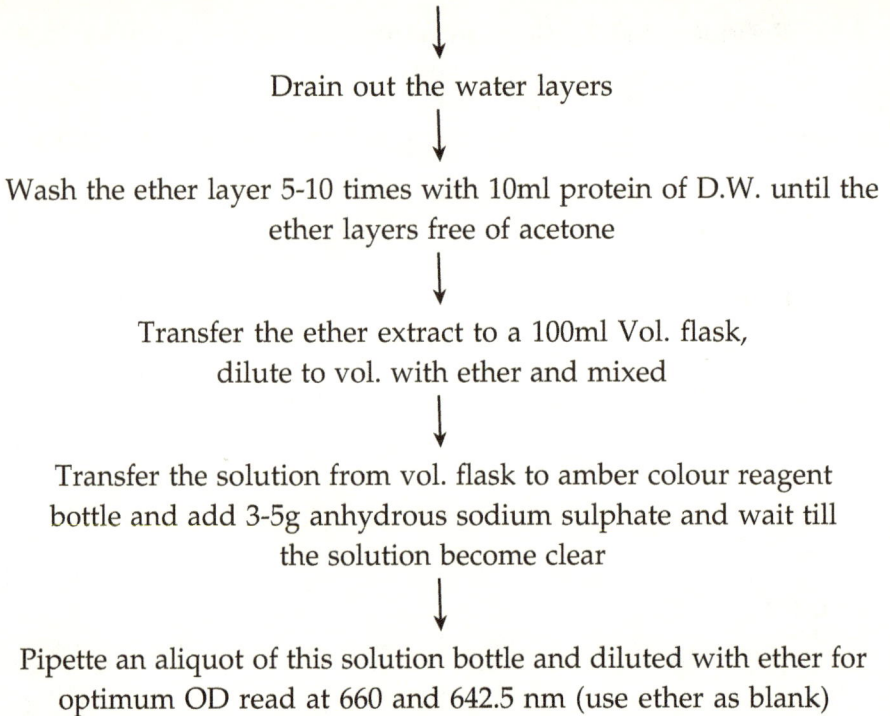

Total Chlorophyll

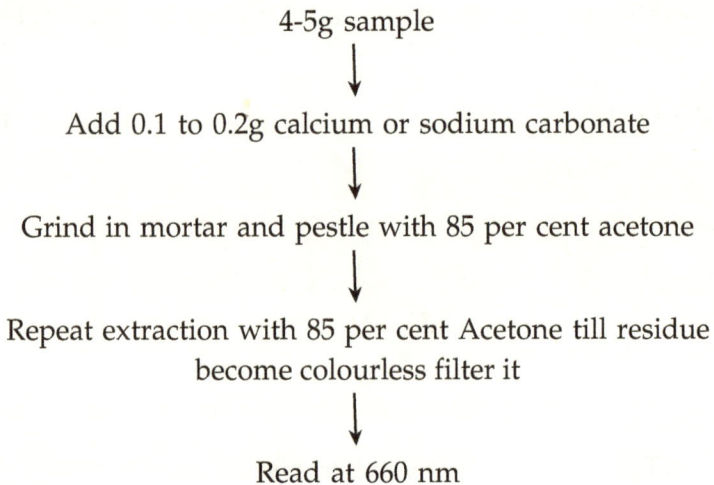

4-5g sample

$\downarrow$

Add 0.1 to 0.2g calcium or sodium carbonate

$\downarrow$

Grind in mortar and pestle with 85 per cent acetone

$\downarrow$

Repeat extraction with 85 per cent Acetone till residue
become colourless filter it

$\downarrow$

Read at 660 nm

Calculation

Total chlorophyll (mg/L) = (7.12xOD at 660nm)+(16.8xOD at
642.5nm)

Chlorophyll a. (mg/L) = (9.93 x OD at 660nm) – (0.777 x OD at 642.5)

Chlorophyll b. (mg/L) = (17.6xOD at 642.5nm) – (2.81 x OD at 660nm)

Precautions

The amount of tissue taken for extraction may be varied. Accordingly amount of 80 per cent acetone used may be altered so that final extract has a volume based on 10mg plant material extracted in 1 ml of acetone.

Reference

Handbook of Analysis and Quality Control for Fruit and Vegetable Products. Second edition (1986) By-S. Ranganna, Tata Mc Graw-Hill Publishing Company Limited, New Delhi. pp. 91-93.

4

Determination of Carotene (Vitamin A)

Principle

Carotenoids the tetraterpenoid (40) compounds are ubiquitous in plants. These terpenoids existing as hydrocarbons (carotenes) or oxygenated derivatives are accessory pigments in photosynthetic system and give colour to plant parts. The total carotenoids are extracted and partitioned in organic solvents on the basis of their solubility. The separation of individual components is effected by chromatography on activated magnesia.

Reagent

1. Acetone
2. Petroleum ether
3. Anhydrous sodium sulphate (Na_2SO_4)
4. Adsorbent : Mix intimately one part by wt. of magnesium oxide (MgO) *i.e.* activated magnesia with three parts of supercel (Hyflosupercell)
5. Eluent : 3 per cent acetone in petroleum ether.

Standard Curve

25mg of β-carotene dissolved in 2.5ml Chloroform and make up with 250 ml of Petroleum ether (stock) [1 ml = 0.1 mg/100μg.

↓

Dilute 1-10 with petroleum ether (10ml to 100ml)

↓

Pipette out 5, 10, 15, 20, 25 and 20 ml of this solution In 100ml of Vol. flask (each containing 3 ml of acetone) [0.5 to 3.0 μg/ml conc.]

↓

Vol made up to 100ml with petroleum ether

↓

OD at 452 nm (using 3 per cent Acetone in petroleum ether as blank)

↓

Plot Abs. against Conc.

Extraction

Weight 5-25g of sample (10-500μg carotene)
(if sample have high sugar it will washed with water on fritted glass funnel under suction)

↓

Grind it in a morter and pestle with adding acetone by using pure sand

↓

Filter through a wad of cotton in to a conical flask and continue extraction and filter till residue colourless

↓

Transfer the filtrate to a separating funnel

↓

Add 10-15 ml petroleum ether

↓

Transfer the pigments in to the petroleum ether phase by diluting the acetone with water or water containing 5 per cent sodium sulphate

↓

Repeat the extraction of the acetone phase with small volumes of petroleum ether till extraction

↓

Filter the petroleum ether through anhydrous sodium sulphate

↓

Concentrate the petroleum ether extract and volume made up to 25 ml

Chromatographic Separation

Preparation of Column

Attach the adsorption tube to a Buchner flask and place a plug of non absorbent cotton in to constriction

↓

Apply vacuum and enough adsorbent to make the column 2-2.5cm in length

↓

Press downs the adsorbent once or twice with a plunger

↓

Loosen the surface of the adsorbent around the edges with a thin edged spatula

↓

Add more adsorbent and repeat the steps until the column is approximately 10 cm in length

↓

Place 1 cm of Sodium sulphate and over the top of the column

Adsorption of Elution

Wet the column by washing with 25-50ml of petroleum ether

↓

While the last ml of the petroleum ether is still above the sodium sulphate. Disconnect the vaccum and transfer the adsorption column to a clean dry Buchner flask

$$\downarrow$$

Pipette out 5-10 ml aliquot of the extract to be chromatographed on to the column and apply suction

$$\downarrow$$

Wash the column continuously with eluent

$$\downarrow$$

Add successive protions of the eluent when the preceding one is just barely visible above the sodium sulphate (Na_2SO_4)

$$\downarrow$$

β-carotene moves of the column prior to till other pigments

$$\downarrow$$

Continue the washing until the desired pigments have moved off the column and the eluent is colourless

$$\downarrow$$

Transfer the contents of flask to a volumetric flask (100 ml) and dilute to volume with eluent

$$\downarrow$$

Read at 452 nm using 3 per cent acetone in petroleum ether as blank

Calculation

$$\mu g\ of\ carotene/100g = \frac{Conc.\ of\ carotene\ in\ solution\ as\ read\ from\ standard\ curve\ (\mu g\ ml) \times Final\ volume \times Dilution \times 100}{Wt.\ of\ the\ sample}$$

Precautions

1. Extraction on carotene should be done very carefully.
2. Chromatographic separation process should be done slowly and accurately.

Reference

Handbook of Analysis and Quality Control for Fruit and Vegetable Products. Second edition (1986) By-S. Ranganna, Tata Mc Graw-Hill Publishing Company Limited, New Delhi. pp. 84-86.

5

Separation and Determination of Carotenoids

Extraction

Total carotenoid from citrus peel or juice can be extracted with Acetone after first removing much of the water by precipitating the colour containing pulp with methanol

↓

Add 200ml of methanol and 15g celite

↓

Filter on Buchner funnel

↓

Place the residue in a warring blender with another 100ml of Acetone

↓

After blending for 1 minute filter and collect the filtrate

↓

Repeat the extraction with acetone till colourless particles

Separation

Combine the filterate to 1 litre separating funnel and 50ml hexane

↓

Add water till layers separate

↓

Drain and discard the aqueous acetone layer

↓

Wash the hexane layer twice with water

↓

Decant the coloured hexane solution in to a 100ml vol. flask and made to volume with hexane

For peel or rag, add 100 ml of methanol to 50g of finely cut material. Blend and decant the aqueous methanol. Extract the residue with Acetone and transfer pigments to hexane as with juice

↓

Determine the absorbance at 450 nm and use β-carotene as a standard as described in following section

Chromatographic Separation

Pack a mixture made of equal wt. of activated magnesia (MgO) and Hyflosupercel in 22x175mm chromatographic column with a glass wool plug and a stopcock at the bottom

↓

Attach it to a vacuum flask

↓

Fill the tube with adsorbent

↓

Apply full vacuum with a water aspirator pump

↓

Use a flat instrument to lamp the adsorbent

↓

Final height of the packed adsorbent should be 10cm.

↓

Place 1 cm layer of anhydrous calcium sulphate on top of the adsorbent

↓

Vacuum is applied on flask to which the column is
attached to shorten elution

↓

Place 25-50 ml of the pigment extract on to the column

↓

As soon as the sample enters the sodium sulphate layer. Elute the
pigments with a sodium of 5 per cent of acetone in hexane

↓

Continue elution until the layer separate the first two coloured band
exit the column

↓

Collect the eluate the each band in separate flasks and dilute each to an
appropriate volume depending on the colour intensity

↓

Elute the remainder of the colour on the column with 50 per cent
acetone in hexane and dilute it with an appropriate volume of hexane.
The final proportion of acetone should be about 25 per cent

Colour Measurement

OD of these solution taken with SP-21 at 450 nm

Standards

10mg of β-carotene to the nearest 0.1 mg

↓

Dissolve it in 100ml of 10 per cent acetone in hexane to make a 10mg/
100ml stock solution

↓

Dilute 20ml of the stock solution to 100m with a same solvent to make the primary standard containing 2mg 100ml

$\downarrow$

Dilute this primary standards with a same solvent to a series of working st. containing between 0.02 to 0.10 mg/100ml in 0.02mg/100ml increments. Construct the standard curve and compare the absorbance of the sample to that of the standard to determine the amount of carotenoids as β-carotene in sample in either 100ml of juice in 100g of sample

Reference

Citrus Fruits and their Production: Analysis and Technology, By S.V. Ting and Russell L. Rouseff (1986). Marcel Dekker Inc. New York, pp. 73-76.

6

Estimation of Total Soluble Sugar

Principle

Simple sugar oligosaccharide, polysaccharides and their derivatives give stable yellow colour when treated with phenol and concentrated H_2SO_4. The absorbance of the colour complex was measured at 490 nm in a spectrophotometer.

Reagent

1. 5 per cent aqueous solution of phenol (Distilled)
2. H_2SO_4 AR grade 96 per cent, specific gravity 1.84

Extraction

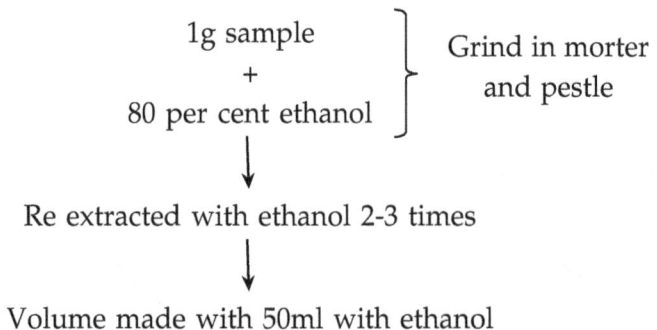

1g sample
+
80 per cent ethanol } Grind in morter and pestle

↓

Re extracted with ethanol 2-3 times

↓

Volume made with 50ml with ethanol

↓

Refluxed for 1 hour on a boiling water bath and filter it

↓

Final volume made up to 50ml/100ml with ethanol

Procedure

Aliquot 1.0ml/2.0ml ⎫
+   ⎬ total volume
D.W. 2/1 ml   ⎭   3 ml

↓

1 per cent, 1ml distilled phenol was added

↓

Mixed well

↓

Add 5 ml conc. H_2SO_4

↓

Kept for 30 min. at room temperature for colour development

↓

Read at 490 nm by SP-21

↓

Standard solution: 100mg/100 ml glucose

↓

1-10 dilution

0.5 to 2.5 ml glucose + D.W. = 3 m + 1ml
1 per cent phenol + 5 ml $H_{-2}SO_4$

↓

Kept for 30 min

↓

Read at 490 nm

Calculation

$$\frac{g}{100\,g} = \frac{G.F. \times O.D. \times Total\ volume}{Aliquot\ taken \times Wt.\ of\ sample \times 10000}$$

Precautions

1. Extrication procedure of total soluble sugar should be done very accurately.
2. Reflection procedure time maintain at least 1 hr. for complete extrication of sugar.

References

Dubois, M; K.A. Gillies; J.K. Hamilton; P.A. Rober, F. Smith (1956). Colorimetric methods of determination of sugars and related substances. *Anal. Chem.* 350-356.

Book: Sadshivam, S. and Manikam, A. (1992). *Biochemical Methods for Agricultural Sciences*, Wiley Eastern Limited, New Delhi.

7

Estimation of Reducing Sugar

Principle

Sugars with reducing property (arising out of the presence of potential aldehyde or keto group). The reducing sugars when heated with alkaline copper tartrate the copper from the cupric to cuprous state and thus cuprous oxide is formed, when cuprous oxide is treated with arsenomolybdic acid the reduction of molybdic acid to molybdenum blue takes place. The blue colour developed absorbs maximally at 540nm.

Reagents

A. Alkaline Copper Reagent

1. 4.0 g copper sulphate
2. 24.0 g Na_2CO_3 anhydrous
3. 12.0 g sodium potassium tartarate   Dissolved in 1 Lit. D.W.
4. 16.0 g sodium bicarbonate
5. 180.0 g Anhydrous sodium sulphate (Mol. Wt. 142.04)

B. Arsenomolybdate Reagent

1. 50.0 g Ammonium molybdate
   (mol. Wt. 1235.90)

2. 42 ml H_2SO_4 AR   } dissolved in
                                                   1 lit. D.W. and
3. 6.0 g Sodium Arsenate (Mol. wt. 312.02)   kept for 2 days
   (disodium hydrogen arsenate)   and filter

Extraction

0.5 to 1.0g sample/50ml Ethanol

(Grind in mortar and pestle → centrifuged in 3000 rpm for 10 min.)

Assay

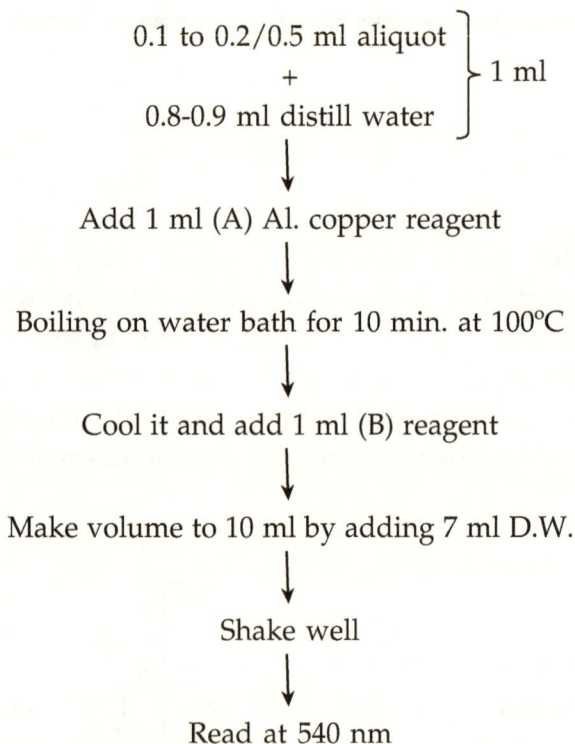

0.1 to 0.2/0.5 ml aliquot
        +   } 1 ml
0.8-0.9 ml distill water

↓

Add 1 ml (A) Al. copper reagent

↓

Boiling on water bath for 10 min. at 100°C

↓

Cool it and add 1 ml (B) reagent

↓

Make volume to 10 ml by adding 7 ml D.W.

↓

Shake well

↓

Read at 540 nm

Calculation

$$\frac{G}{100}g = O.D. \times \frac{G.F.(152)}{\text{Aliquot}} \times \frac{\text{Total volume (50 ml)}}{\text{Sample wt.} \times 10000}$$
$$(0.1-0.5\,ml)$$

Precautions

Alkaline copper reagent and arsenomolybdate reagent preparation procedure must watch very carefully.

Reference

Sadashivam, S. and Manikam, A. (1992): *Biochemical Methods for Agricultural Sciences*, Wiley Eastern Limited New Delhi.

8
Determination of Total Phenols

Phenols

The aromatic compounds with hydroxyl groups are widespread in plant kingdom. Resistance to diseases and pests is due to this. Phenols include an array of compounds like tannins, flavonols. etc.

Principle

Phenols react with phosphomolydic acid in Folin Ciocalteau reagent in alkaline medium and produce coloured complex (molybdenum blue).

Reagents

1. Folin-ciocalteau reagent (phenol reagent) 1 : 1 D.W.
2. 20 per cent Na_2CO_3

Procedure

1 ml tissue were grind in 25 ml 80 per cent methanol in morter and pestle and

Filter it

↓

$$\left.\begin{array}{c} 0.1/0.2 \text{ ml aliquot} \\ + \\ 0.9/0.3 \text{ ml D.W.} \end{array}\right\} 1 \text{ ml}$$

↓

Add 1 ml phenol reagent

↓

Add 2 ml 20 per cent Na_2CO_3

↓

Boil at 100°C for 1-2 min.

↓

Cool it

↓

Volume made up 10 ml with D.W.

↓

Centrifuged it and read at 650 nm by SP-21

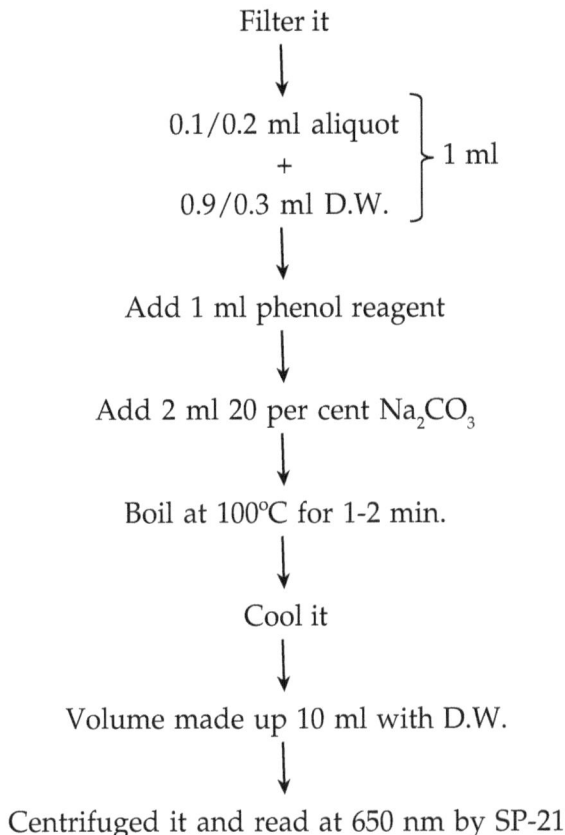

Standard Curve

10 mg catechol/100ml D.W.

Conc. 10 µg/ml

0.1 ml (10 µg) + 0.9ml D.W. + 1ml Phenol reagent 1:1 +

2ml 20 per cent Na_2CO_3

0.2 ml (20 µg) + 0.8ml D.W.   ↓

0.3 ml (30 µg) + 0.7ml D.W.   Boil it 100°C

0.4 ml (40 µg) + 0.6ml D.W.   ↓

0.5 ml (50 µg) + 0.5ml D.W.   Cool it

↓

Volume made up to 10 ml

↓

Centrifuged it

$\downarrow$

Read at 650 nm

Calculation

$$\frac{g}{100\,g} = \frac{G.F. \times O.D. \times Total\ volume}{Aliquot\ taken \times Wt.\ of\ sample \times 10000}$$

Precautions

1. Folin – ciocaltaeue reagent prepared freshly.

2. $NaCO_3$ must be dissolved in 0.1 N NaOH for making complete saturated solution.

Reference

Bray, H.G. and Thorpe, W.V. (1954) Analysis of phenolic compounds of interest in metabolism. *Methods in Biochemical Analysis*. 1 : 27-37.

9

Estimation of True Protein by Folin – Lowry's Method

Principle

The blue colour developed by the reduction of the phosphomolybdic-phosphotungstic compontents in the Folin-Ciocalteau reagent by the amino acids tyrosine and tryptophan present in the protein. Plus the colour developed by the biuret reaction of the protein with the alkaline cupric tartrate are measured in the Lowry's method.

Reagents

1. 2 per cent Na_2CO_3 in 0.1 N NaOH
2. 0.5 per cent $CuSO_4$ is 1 per cent Sodium Potassium Tartarate
3. Folin –ciocalteau (Phenol reagent) 1:1 D.W.
4. Bovine Serum Albumin (BSA) 0.2 mg/ml in 0.1 NaOH
5. Mix reagent 1 and 2, 50:1 before assay

Procedure

$$0.2 \text{ ml Aliquot} \atop + \atop 2.8 \text{ ml D.W.} \Big\} \quad \begin{array}{c} 3 \text{ ml total volume} \\ \text{adjusted} \end{array}$$

↓

5 ml reagent (No. 5)

↓

Add 0.5 ml Folin ciocalteau (1.1 reagent)

↓

Vortex

↓

Kept for 30 min. at 25°C for colour development

↓

Bluish colour development

↓

Read at 750nm by SP-21

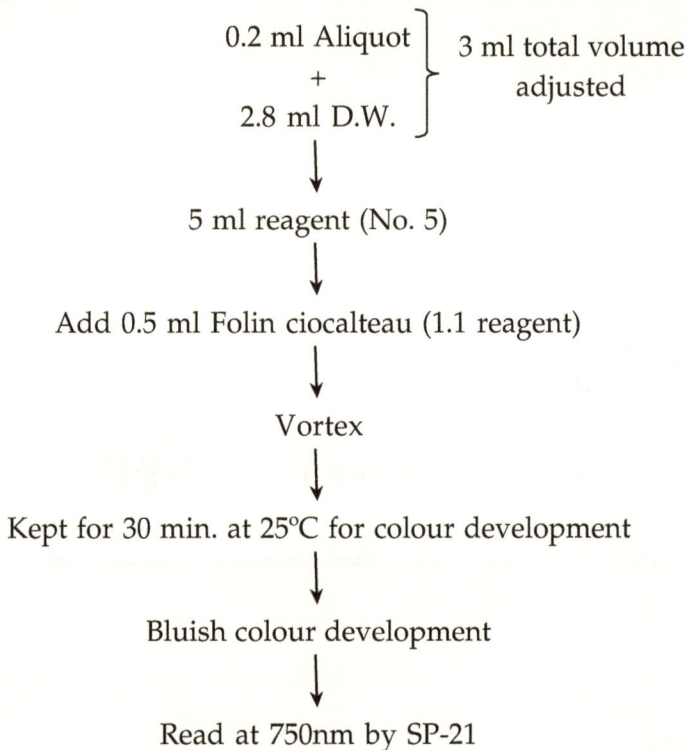

Standard Curve

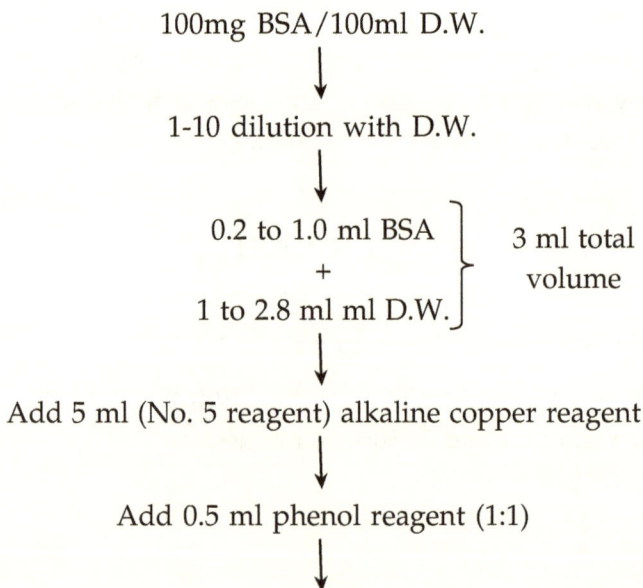

100mg BSA/100ml D.W.

↓

1-10 dilution with D.W.

↓

$$0.2 \text{ to } 1.0 \text{ ml BSA} \atop + \atop 1 \text{ to } 2.8 \text{ ml ml D.W.} \Big\} \quad \begin{array}{c} 3 \text{ ml total} \\ \text{volume} \end{array}$$

↓

Add 5 ml (No. 5 reagent) alkaline copper reagent

↓

Add 0.5 ml phenol reagent (1:1)

↓

Vortex

↓

Kept for 30 min for colour development

↓

Read O.D. at 750 nm

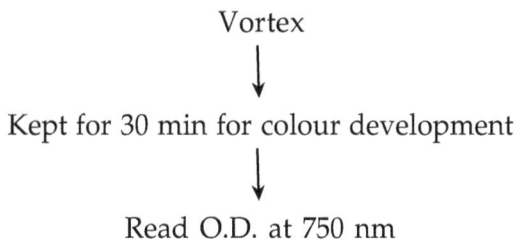

Express results as protein mg/g on fresh weight basis

Calculation

$$\frac{g}{100\,g} = \frac{G.F. \times O.D. \times Total\ volume}{Aliquot\ taken \times Wt.\ of\ sample \times 10000}$$

Precautions

1. During preparation of $CuSO_4$ reagent no precipited solution should be observed.

2. Standard solution of BSA should be prepared very carefully.

References

Lowry, O.H., Rosebrough, N.J., Farr, A.L. and Randall, R.J. (1951). Protein measurement with the folin phenol reagent. J. Bio. Chem. 193:265.

Book: Sadashivam, S. and Manikam, A. (1992). *Biochemical Methods for Agricultural Sciences*, Wiley Eastern Limited, New Delhi.

10
Determination of Methionine

Principle

Methionine is one of the essential sulphur-containing amino acids. The protein in the grain is first hydrolysed under mild acidic condition. The liberated methionine gives an yellow colour with nitroprusside solution under alkaline condition and truns red on acidification. Glycine is added to the reaction mixture in order to inhibit colour formation with other amino acids.

Methionine content was analyzed as descrbied by Horn *et al*. (1946).

Reagent

1. 6 NHCl
2. 5 N NaOH
3. 1 per cent sodium nitroprusside
4. 3 per cent glycine solution

Procedure

0.5 g sample was weighed and transferred into receiving flask

↓

20 ml of 6N HCl was added to the same flask. The material was refluxed for 20-24 hrs.

↓

After complete reflection the content of the flask was transferred in to China disc it was then evaporated on water bath with the addition of 1g activated charcoal

↓

Evaporation was continued until the content of China disc become viscous

↓

Hot distilled water was added and filter through Whatman filter paper No. the filtrate was collected in 25 ml volumetric flask

↓

The china disk was washed with little amount of hot water and about 5-6 times and washing were collected in the same volumetric flask

↓

Volume was made up to 25 ml.

↓

This hydrolyzate was used for colorimetric estimation of methionine

↓

10ml hydrolyzate extract was transferred to 100ml beaker with the addition of 4ml of distilled water. 2 ml of 5 N NaOH was added to same beaker

↓

Further 0.1 ml of 1 per cent sodium nitroprusside and 2 ml of 3 per cent glycine solution was also added to develop the colour

↓

The intensity of the colour was measured along with the blank on SP-20 at 450nm.

↓

The calculation was done with the help of standard curve of methionine.

Calculation

$$\frac{g}{16gN} = \frac{\text{Reading of the sample} \times 150}{\text{Protein \% of the sample}}$$

Precautions

1. Reflection time of methionine exvraction must be 20-24hr. for complet extraction.
2. Colour development procedure should be watch very correctly.

References

Horn, J.M.; Jones D.B. and Blum, A.E. (1946). Colorimetric determination of methionine in protein and foods J. Biol. Chem. 166-313.

Book: Sadashivam, S. and Manikam, A. (1992). *Biochemical Methods for Agricultural Sciences*, Wiley Eastern Limited New Delhi.

11
Estimation of Proline

Principle

Proline is a basic amino acid. During selective extraction with aqueous sulphosalicylic acid, proteins are precipitated as a complex. Other interfering materials are also presumably removed by absorption to the protein-sulphosalicylic acid complex. The extracted proline is made to react with ninhydrin in acidic condition (pH 1.0) to from the chromophore (red colour) and read as 520nm.

Reagent

25 g nin-hydrine was dissolved in 30ml glacial acetic acid and 20ml of 6N orthophosphoric acid with continuos stirring until dissolved and stored at low temperature before the use (stable for 24 hours).

Procedure

200mg of well ground seed sample was homogenized thoroughly with 10ml of reagent and sulphosalic acid and centrifuged at 400rpm for 20 minute

↓

2 ml of supernatant was mixed well with 2 ml of acid nin-hydrine and 2 ml acetic acid.

$\downarrow$

Kept the tubes on boiling water bath for 1 hr. after the reaction was
terminated by placing the tube in acid box.

$\downarrow$

The reaction mixture was then shaken for vigorously with 4 ml toluene
and kept for several hrs. at room temperature.

$\downarrow$

The colour intensity was measured at 520 nm on SP-20.
Toluene was used as blank. The standard curve of DL-proline
was also prepared simultaneously.

Precautions

1. 6N orthophosphoric acid solution prepared very accurately.

2. Toluene layer must be removed very carefully.

References

Bates, L.S.; Walderen, R.P. and Teare, I.D. (1973). Rapid determination of
free proline for water stress studies. *Plant and Soil* 39:205-208.

Book: Sadashivam, S. and Manikam, A. (1992). *Biochemical Methods for
Agricultural Sciences*, Wiley Eastern Limited, New Delhi.

12

Determination of Tryptophan

Principle

The indole ring of tryphophan gives an orange-red colour with ferric chloride under strong acidic conditions which is measurable by SP-21 at 545nm.

Tryptophan content was estimated by the method of Spies and Camber (1949).

Reagent

1. 19N H_2SO_4
2. p-dimethyl amino benzyldehyde
3. 0.045 per cent sodium nitrate

Procedure

0.2 g or (50 mg) homogenous sample was transferred into a 100 ml conical flask and 10 ml 19N H_2SO_4 was also added

↓

The content of conical flask were kept for 12 hrs. in dark

↓

After expiry of period 1 ml distill water, 1 ml P-dimethyl amino benzyldehyde (0.3 per cent in 2N H_2SO_4) and 0.1 ml sodium nitrate (0.045 per cent) was added

$$\downarrow$$

This was kept for 30 min.

$$\downarrow$$

The intensity of the colour was measured with the help of SP-21 at 545 nm. The calculation were done by standard curve of tryptophan.

Calculation

0.34 st O.D. contain = 0.1 mg tryptophan

$$\text{Sample O.D. (0.21) contain} = 0.1 \times \frac{0.21}{0.34} = \text{X value (0.0617)}$$

25 mg sample contain = X value

$$100 \text{ mg sample contain} = \frac{X}{25} \times 100 = \text{2X value (0.247)}$$

Suppose 30g protein = 2X

$$100 \text{ g protein} = \frac{2x}{30} \times 100 = \text{g/16g N (0.823)}$$

Precautions

1. 19 N solution of H_2SO_4 must be prepared very correctly.

References

Spies, J.T. and Camber, D.C. (1949). Chemical determination of Tryptophan in protein. *Anal. Chem.* 21:1249.

Book: Sadashivam, S. and Manikam, A. (1992). *Biochemical Methods for Agricultural Sciences*, Wiley Eastern Limited, New Delhi.

13

Estimation of Pectin Substances

Principle

Pectin extracted from the plant material is sponified with alkali and precipitated a s calcium pectate from an acid solution by the addition of calcium chloride. The calcium pectate precipitate is washed until free from chloride dried and weight.

Reagents

1. 1 N acetic acid (approximate) : dilute 30 ml of glacial acetic acid to 500 ml D.W.

2. 1 N calcium chloride Anhydrous : Dissolve 27.5g of Anhydrous Calcium chloride in D.W. dilute to 500 ml

3. 1 per cent silver nitrate : Dissolve 1g of $AgNO_3$ in 100 ml D.W.

4. $0.005 \text{ N HCl} = \dfrac{\text{eq. wt.} \times N \times 100}{\text{Sp. gravity} \times \text{Purity}} =$

$$\dfrac{36.5 \times 0.005 \times 100}{1.18 \times 35.4} = 4.368 \text{ ml per lit.}$$

5. 1 N NaOH

Procedure

Wt. 50g blended sample in to 1000 ml beaker

↓

Extract with 400ml 0.05 N HCl for 2 hr. at 80-90°C

↓

Cool, filter through watman No. 4 and make up 500 ml

↓

Repeated extraction of pulped vegetables or fruits in cold water followed by boiling and mixed extract prior to filtration or boiling the pulped material with water without any addition of acid

↓

To stabilize the insoluble protein, acid extraction is considered essential

Alternate Procedure of Acid Extraction

Biol initially with 0.01 N HCl for 30 min.

↓

Filter under sustain and wash the residue with hot water

↓

To residue add 0.05 N HCl boil of 20 min. and filter as before

↓

To the residue and 0.3 N HCl, boil for 10 min and filter

↓

Combine the filtrates, cool and make up to volume

↓

Dried pectin extracted and purified as before may also be used

↓

Wt. 200mg of dried pectin in to 100ml beaker

↓

Wet with 2 or 3 ml of alcohol

↓

Add 400ml of D.W. with stirring

↓

Heat to boiling and cool

↓

Transfer to a 500ml volumetric flask and make upto volumetric after filter (Whatman filter paper No. 4)

PECTIC SUBSTANCES

Pectic substances is juices can be determined as Calcium pectate

PPt. 25-50 ml of the juice with four volumes of acidified alcohol (5 ml HCl/lit.)

↓

Allow to stand for 30 min.

↓

Centrifuge the mixture as discard the supernatant

↓

Wash the precipitate with 100-150ml of 75 per cent alcohol and dissolved in 50ml water

↓

If pectin content is more, make up to a known volume and take 50ml

↓

Proceed further by neutralizing the acid with 1 N NaOH as given under the procedure to the estimation of pectin as calcium pectate

↓

The pectin content in precipitate was also be determined by the colorimetric method

↓

Pipette 100-200 ml aliquot each in to 1000 ml beaker

↓

Add 250 ml D.W.

↓

Neutralize the acid with 1 N NaOH using phenopthalein as indicator

↓

Pipette 10ml of 1 N NaOH in excess with constant stirring

↓

Allow to stand over night

↓

Then add 50 ml of 1 N Acetic acid and after 5 min.

↓

Add 25ml of 1 N calcium chloride solution with stirring
After allowing it to stand for 1 hr. boil for 1-2 min.

↓

Filter through Whatman filter paper No. 2
(Wt. with water dry in over at 102°C for 2 hrs.)

↓

Cool in a desiccator and weight in covered dish

↓

Wash the precipitate with water which is almost boiling
until free form chlorides

↓

Test using $AgNO_3$

↓

Transfer the filter paper containing Calcium pectate to the original
weighing dish, dry overnight at 100°C

Calculation

$$\% \text{ Calcium pectate} = \frac{\text{Wt. of calcium pectate (Total volume)} \times 500 \times 100}{\text{ml. of filtrate taken for estimation} \times \text{Wt. of sample}}$$

Precautions

1. Ag NO_3 solution must be prepared very accurately.
2. Weighing process should be done very accurately.

Reference

Handbook of Analysis and Quality Control for Fruit and Vegetable Products. Second edition (1986) By-S. Ranganna, Tata Mc Graw-Hill Publishing Company Limited, New Delhi. pp. 40-42.

14

Determination of Furfural

Principle

Ascorbic acid as well as pentose sugar give rise to furfual when may polymerize or combine with amino compounds to cause non-enzymatic browning in fruit and vegetables products. The measurement of furfural therefore, is of value is the study of non-enzymatic browning in storage studies. It may be measured by making use of its absorption maximum in the UV at 227 nm or by its colour reaction with aniline and HCl.

Spectropholometric Method

Reagent

furfural Standard solution weight 1 ml of redistilled furfural in to a 100 ml volumetric flask and make up to mark with alcohol.

When required, dilute 5ml to 500 ml with 50 per cent alcohol (conc. is 116 mg/lit.)

Procedure

Liquid samples: If the solid content is 25g/100 ml or less add.

12.5-25 ml of water

$\downarrow$

If the solvent content is more than 25g/100ml, add 5 ml of D.W. for each of 10g of solid matter present. Add sufficient alcohol to raise the conc. to 50 per cent

$\downarrow$

Mix and filter

$\downarrow$

Pipette 100-200ml of the filtrate, stem distil slowly, collecting volume of distillate equal to that of volume taken for distillation

$\downarrow$

Dilute the distillate with known volume of 50 per cent alcohol and determine absorbance at 277nm

$\downarrow$

Determine the absorbance of standard solutions of furfural containing 0, 1, 2, 3, 4 and 5mg of furfural per lit.

$\downarrow$

Plot standard curve against abs. and read once in sample for the curve

Calculation

$$\text{Furfural mg}\% = \frac{\text{mg of furfural} \times \text{Dilution} \times 100}{\text{Wt. or volume of sample} \times 100}$$

Colorimetric Method

Prepare standard furfural solution as in spectrophotometer method

$\downarrow$

Pipette aliquot (0, 5, 1, 2, 3, 4 and 5 ml) of the std. (116 mg/lit.) furfural solution to a 50 ml graduated cylinders and make up to mark with 50 per cent ethyl alcohol

$\downarrow$

Add 2 ml of colourless aniline and 0.5 ml HCl

↓

Keep for 15 min and measure the colour at 520 nm
(Light pink colour formed)

↓

Measure the furfural content in the sample (5 ml) dilute an aliquot of the distillate to 50 ml with 50 per cent ethyl alcohol

↓

Develop and measures the colour as in the std.

In the colorimetric method reproducible results are obtained only at constant alcohol content. In the UV method, alcohol conc. has no effect on the determination.

Precautions

Furfural standard must be prepared very accurately.

References

Schoeneman, R.L. (1960) J. Ass of Agric. Chemistry, 43, 657, 6. Stilling, R.A. and B.L. Browning. *Ind. Eng. Chem. and Ed.* 12, 499 (1940).

Handbook of Analysis and Quality Control for Fruit and Vegetable Products. Second edition (1986). By-S. Ranganna, Tata Mc Graw-Hill Publishing Company Limited, New Delhi. pp. 891-892.

15

Determination of Stevens Clouds Stability Test

Reagents

1.

3g pectin (rapid set)

↓

Add few drops of alcohol

↓

Make 100ml vol with warm distilled water
(use stirrer for proper mixing)

2. Sodium benzoate – 4.4g/100ml D.W.

3. Barium chloride – 30g/100ml D.W.

4. Citric acid – 50g/100ml D.W.

Procedure

90 or 45 ml juice single strength in 250 ml beaker

↓

Add 3.6 or 1.8 ml of pectin

↓

Add 1.3 or 0.65ml barium chloride solution

↓

Add 0.5 or 0.25 ml sodium benzoate

↓

Adjust the pH 3.1 to 3.2 with citric acid in case of orange (pH around 4.3) or 0.1 N NaOH for lime and lemon

↓

Mixed well, transfer to a clear screw cap of bottle

↓

Incubate at 48.3° to 48.9°C for 5 days

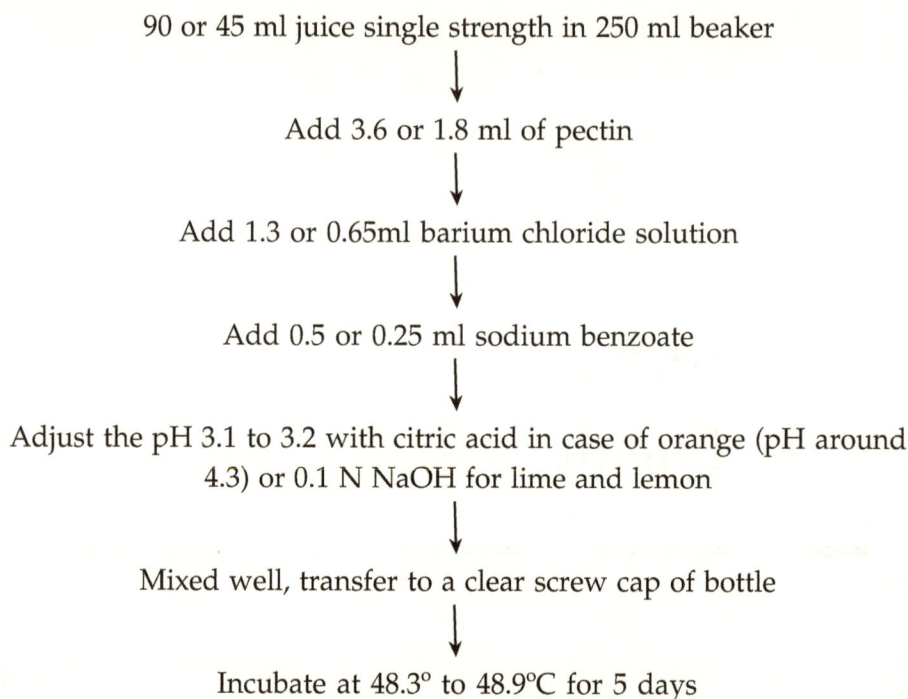

Interpretation

Examine the sample during and after incubation for signs of separation, flouation or clarification. The absence of these conditions indicates a negative test for residual activity, dilute a portion of the test sample with an equal volume of water and centrifuge in 15 ml tubes at 2000 rpm (16 inch diameter centrifuge) for 2 min. The supermatant liquid following centrifugation should remain good cloud. A clear scrum after centrifugs in indicative of enzyme action.

Precautions

1. Barium chloride solution must be prepared very accurately.
2. Interpretation of test must be done carefully.

Reference

Handbook of Analysis and Quality Control for Fruit and Vegetable Products. Second edition (1986). By-S. Ranganna, Tata Mc Graw-Hill Publishing Company Limited, New Delhi. pp. 918-919.

16
Determination of Ethanol

Principle

ADH
1. Ethanol + NAD $\longrightarrow$ acetaldehyde + NADH + H

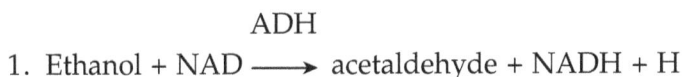

AIDH
2. Acetaldehyde + NAD + $H_2O \longrightarrow$ Acetate – NAOH + H

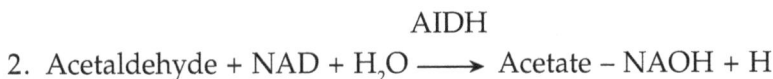

Reagents

1. Potassium diphosphate solution ($K_4P_2O_7$, 0.30 mol/L pH 9.0)

    Dissove 5.0g $K_4P_2O_7$ with Ca, 40 ml water, adjust to pH 9.0 with HCl, 1 mol/L and made up to 50 ml with water.

2. Nicotinamide-adenine dinuoleotide (β-NAD, 49m mol/L); dissolve 103 mg (β-NAD, free acid with 3 ml water.

3. Aldehyde dehydrogenesen (75 KU)

    (Dissolve that amount of AIDH preparation (from yeast, lyophilized, stabilized with potassium phosphate) with corresponds to 40U. lyophilized enzyme preparation (at 25°C, acetaldehyde as substrate) with 0.5 ml water.

4. Alcohol dehydrogenase (ca 900 KU/L)

   Use the stock suspension of ADH (from yeast suspended in ammonium sulphate solution, 3.2 mol/L, pH 6.0≥300U/mg protein at 25°C, ethanol as substrate undiluted.

5. Perchloric acid (0.33 mol/L)

   Dilute 2.85 ml perohloric acid, sp gr, 1.67, 70 per cent W/W to 100ml with water.

6. Perchloric acid (1 mol/L)

   Dilute 8.64 ml perchloric acid sp. Gr. 1.67, 70 per cent, W/W to 100 ml with water.

Sample Preparation

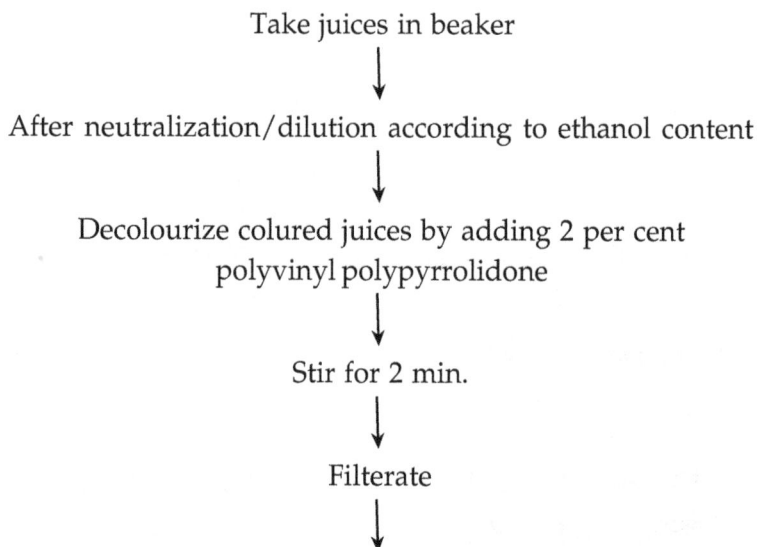

Take juices in beaker

↓

After neutralization/dilution according to ethanol content

↓

Decolourize colured juices by adding 2 per cent
polyvinyl polypyrrolidone

↓

Stir for 2 min.

↓

Filterate

↓

Use clean solution for the assay after neutralization and dilution

Assay Condition

Wavelength Hg 334, 339 or Hg 365 nm light path 10mm final volume 2.64 ml, room temp, measurement against air

A reagent blank with water instead of sample is essential because of impurities of alcohol in the reagents.

Measurement			
Pipette Successively in to the Cuvette	*Reagent Blank*	*Sample*	*Concentration in Assy Mixture*
Potassium diphosphate solution (1)	1.0ml	1.0 ml	$K_4P_2O_7$ 114 mmol/l
NAD solution (2)	0.10 ml	0.10 ml	NAD 1.86 mmol/l
Sample	—	0.10ml	Ethanol upto 80μ mol/l
AIDH solution (3)	0.02 ml	0.02 ml	AIDH 568 U/l
Water	1.50 ml	1.40 ml	
Mix after 2 min read absorption of the solution (A1)			
ADH (4)	0.02 ml	0.02 ml	ADH 68 KU/L

Mix on completion of reaction (ca 6-8 min). Read absorption of the solution (A2) immediately one after the others.

Calculation

Correct the absorbence difference (A2-A1) of sample for the absorbance difference of reagent blank, yielding Δ A. According to eqn. (b) and (b1) and considering that 1 mole ethanol corresponds to 2 moles of NADH, *viz* the conc. of ethanol in the sample solution is (mol. wt. 46.07).

	Hg 334 nm	*339nm*	*Hg365nm*
C=	ΔA x 2.136	ΔA x 2.095	ΔA x 3.882 mmol/L
P=	ΔA x 98.40	ΔA x 96.53	ΔA x 1.78 mg/L

The result must be multiplied by the appropriate factor of the sample has been deprotenized neutralized or diluted in any way.

Precautions

Alcohol dehydrosenase and aldehyde dehydrogenase solution should be prepared very accurately.

References

Hans-Otto-Beutles (reprint) pp. 598-606.

Chap. 4.1, Two and One carbon compound.

17
Determination of Acetaldehyde (CH₃CHO)

Principle

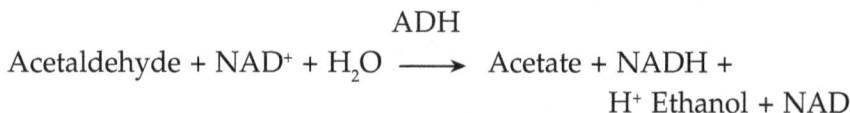

$$\text{Acetaldehyde} + \text{NAD}^+ + \text{H}_2\text{O} \xrightarrow{\text{ADH}} \text{Acetate} + \text{NADH} + \text{H}^+ \text{Ethanol} + \text{NAD}$$

Reagent

1. Potassium diphosphate solution ($K_4P_2O_7$ with Ca 40 ml water adjust to pH 9.0 with HCl. 1 mol/L and makeup to 50ml with water.

2. β-NAD (Nicotinamide adenine dinucleotide 49 mol/L): dissolve 103mg. β-NAD, free acid with 3 ml water.

3. Aldehyde dehydrogenase (AIDH, 75 KU/I)

   Dissolve that amount of acid preparation (from yeast, lyophilized, stabilized with potassium phosphate) which corresponds to 40 U lyophilized enzyme preparation (at 25°C, acetaldehyde as substrate with 0.5 ml water).

4. Perchloric acid (1.0 mol/L)

   Dilute 8.55 ml perchloric acid, sp. Gr 1.67 70 per cent 9 w/w with water and make up to 100ml

5. Carrez I-solution [(K₄Fe(CN)₆)], 85 mmol/L (Potassium ferrocyanide): Dissolve 3.6g with water and make up 100ml

6. Carrez II solution $ZnSO_4.7H_2O$ (Zinc sulphate, 250mmol/L. Dissolve 7.20g $ZnSO_4$ with water and make up to 100ml

Sample Preparation

Turbit free solution of fruit juice was taken in beaker

$\downarrow$

Dilute so that the acctaldehyde connentration is less than 0.1g/L

$\downarrow$

Use the clear solution for the assay

Standard Solution

200mg freshly distilled acetaldehyde (ca, 260µl) in to 100 ml vol. flask which is approx. half of the full with water. Make up to the mark with water and mix. Store the solution for about 12 hrs. at +4°C before diluting with water in a ratio of 1.9 use 0.1 ml of diluted solution for the assay (= 1.2mg acetaldehyde/ml).

Assay Condition

Wavelength 339, Hg 334 of Hg 365 mm light path 10 min; final volume 3.12 ml; room temp.; measurement against air. A reagent blank with water instead of sample is essential because of small impurities of the reagents with certain aldehydes.

Measurement

Pipette Successively in to the Cuvette	Reagent Blank	Sample	Concentration in Assy Mixture
Potassium diphosphate solution (1)	1.0ml	1.0 ml	$K_4P_2O_7$ 96 mmol/L
NAD solution (2)	0.10 ml	0.10 ml	NAD 1.57 mmol/L
Sample	—	0.10ml	Acetaldehyde up to 140 µ mol/L
Water	2.0ml	1.90ml	

Contd...

Contd...

Pipette Successively in to the Cuvette	Reagent Blank	Sample	Concentration in Assy Mixture
Mix thoroughly with plastic spatula and read absorption (A₁) after 2-3 min.			
AIDH solution (3)	0.02 ml	0.02 ml	ADH 480 U/L
Mix on completion of reaction (ca 3-5 min). Read absorption of the solution (A2).			

Calculation

Calculate the absorbance difference (A2-A1). Use $\Delta A = (A2-A1)$ sample (A2-A1) blank for calculation. According to eqn. (b) and (b1) in formulate, the conc. In the sample is (wt. of acetaldehyce is 44.05 for values.

	Hg 334 nm	339nm	Hg365nm
C=	$\Delta A \times 5.048$	$\Delta A \times 4.952$	$\Delta A \times 9.176$ mmol/L
P=	$\Delta A \times 222.4$	$\Delta A \times 218.1$	$\Delta A \times 404.2$ mg/L

The result must be multiplied by the appropriate factor of the sample has been deprotenized neutralized or diluted in any way.

Precautions

Calculation procedure of aldehyde measurement must be very correctly.

References

Hans-Otto-Beutles (Xerox reprint) pp. 598-606.

Chap. 4.1, Two and One carbon compound.

18

Carotenoids Estimation by HPLC

Principle

This method employs a novel, rapid sample preparation on, separation is achieved through the use of non-aqueous solvent system on a reverse phase (C-18) column. The method employs saponification to simplify the separation and is specific for β-cryptoxanthin and α-carotene.

Equipment

A single high pressure pump capable of pulseless flow, a 25 cm x 4.6 mm i.d. Dupont (Wilington, D.E.) C-18 column, an injector, a variable wavelength detector set at 450nm and an integrator-printer plotters are required for this analysis. A Sorvell Omni-mixture (Newton, CT) with a 6 ml micro attachment is used to extract for cartones. A Baker 10-SPE (Phillipsburgh, N.J.) is used for the sample preparation.

Standard and Reagent

Authentic α and β carotenes are recrystallized from Benzene/Methanol (1:3). β-cryptoxanthin is not commercially available and is isolated from citrus juice using the procedure of Stewart and Wheaton (1971). All solvents used were HPLC grade.

Sample Preparation

A 10 ml of orange juice is centrifuged for 5 min 6000rpm to obtain pellet which contains the carotenoids. The clarified juice is decanted and discarded. Using 2 ml of methanol, pellet is resuspended and recentrifuged. The supernatant liquid is discarded and decanted. Finally an additional 3 ml of methanol is added to the pellet and carotenoids extracted after stirring in the Omni-Mixture for 1 Min at 10°C. The pellet is extracted more times and 9 ml of methanol is saved for saponification.

Saponification and Sample Clean Up

4.5 ml of methanolic KOH (10g/100ml) are added to 9 ml of methanolic carotenoids extract and allow to stand in the dark for 1 hr. The mixture is extracted once with 30 ml of methylene chloride and then washed 4 x20 ml with water. The light yellow organic layer containing the carotenoids is evaporated to dryness under nitrogen. Using 2ml methanol, the residue is redissolved and placed upon at 6 ml C-18 preconditioned column. The column is washed with 4.5 ml of 95.5 (methanol a water V/V) to remove the polar carotenoids and non-polar carotenoids eluted with 3 ml of chloride. The non-polar carotenoid extract is evaporated to dryness and redissolved in the chronathgraphic solvent system just prior to injection.

Chromatographic Condition

The chromatographic solvent system (mobile phase) consisted of acetonitrile : methylene chloride : methanol (65:25:10 v/v). Flow rate was 1.5 ml injection volume was 50 µl.

Analysis time was 20 min. The column was washed periodically with methylene chloride and equilibrated with the mobile phase.

Quantitation

Cartenoid concentrations were determined from the response factor obtained from the respective standards.

Precautions

1. Chromatograthic condition of HPLC must maintain.
2. Degas solvent before use to remove dissolved gases.
3. Use only blunt tipped needle for sample injection.

4. Column should be washed thoroughly after the analysis either in methanol or 0.1 per cent sodium azide to prevent from microbial growth.

Reference

Citrus Fruits and their Production: Analysis and Technology, By S.V. Ting and Russell L. Rouseff (1986). Marcel Dekker Inc. New York, pp. 76-78.

19
Sugar Analysis by HPLC

Principle

The resolving power of chromatographic column increases with column length and the number of a the theoretical plate unit length. The number of theoretical plates is related to the surface area of the stationary phase, the better the resolution, unfortunately the smaller the particle size, the greater is the resistance to flow of mobile phase. This creates a back pressure in the column that is sufficient to damage the matrix structure of the stationary phase, thereby actually reducing elent flow and impairing resolution.

This primary sugars in citrus can be essentially baseline separated and quantified within 20 min.

Equipment

A single HPLC pump capable of delivering pulse free flow and injector are required with the refractive index detector (Water Associated R-40), the refractive index detector, or equivalent at 8X.

The separation is accomplished on an amine column 4.6 mm i.d. x 25 (or 30) cm. Detector stability is greatly improved if this column is insulated. To extend the life of the anabtical column a guard column (Brown lee

Labs amino spheris or equivalent) is highly recommended. A baker-10 solid phase extraction (SPE) system of water associates Sep Pak is used to clean up the samples further preserving the life of the column. An integrator printer plotter is used to record and calculate the data.

Standard

100mg of fructose, glucose and maltose along with 200mg of highly purity sucrose is added to a small vial. The sugar are dissolved of enough distill water (HPLC) grade to bring the total weight to 5g std. are freshly prepared each week.

Sample Preparation

Floating pulp and some suspended solids are removed for the juice using a benchtop centrifuge

↓

Water C_{18} sep pack or baker 10 SPE C_{18} cartridge (6 ml is conditioned by passing 5 ml of methanol (MeOH) followed by 10ml of deionized water

↓

2ml of juice is passed through cash cartriged

↓

Discarded to remove any water which might dilute the sample

↓

3 more ml of juice is passed through each cartriged in to labeled vial

↓

If the juice is excessively turbid it is filtered with a 0.45 ml filter

Chromatographic Condition

Mobile phase consist of HPLC grade acetonitrile and deionized water (75:25 v/v)

↓

Flow rate is 1.0ml/min.

↓

Solvent is degassed daily with sonications and vacuum

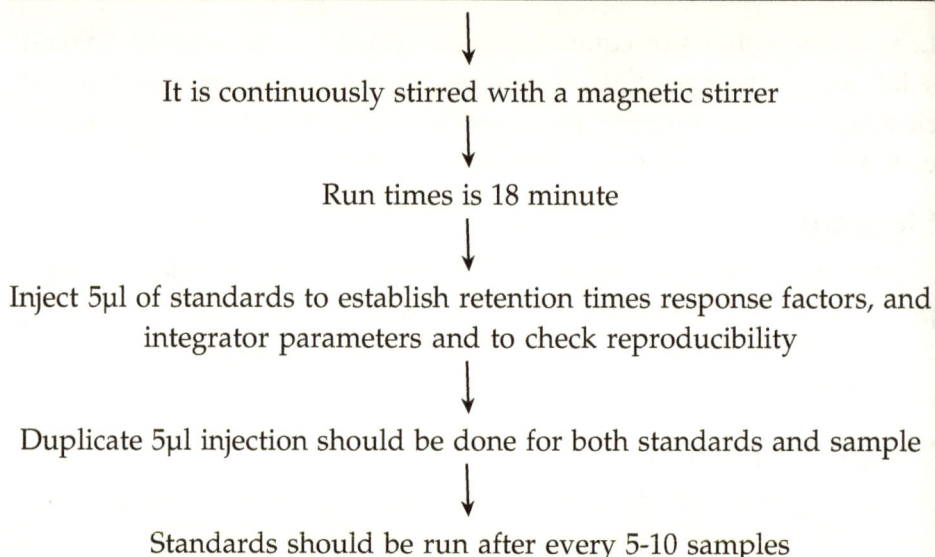

$\downarrow$

It is continuously stirred with a magnetic stirrer

$\downarrow$

Run times is 18 minute

$\downarrow$

Inject 5µl of standards to establish retention times response factors, and integrator parameters and to check reproducibility

$\downarrow$

Duplicate 5µl injection should be done for both standards and sample

$\downarrow$

Standards should be run after every 5-10 samples

Calculation

Individual juice sugar concentration and calculated average peak area values

$$\text{Wt \% sugar} = \text{Wt \% standard} \times \frac{\text{Area (sample)}}{\text{Area (standard)}} \text{ Or}$$

$$\text{Wt \% sugar} = \frac{\text{Area (sample)}}{\text{KF}}$$

where,

$$\text{KF} = \text{Concentration factor} \times \frac{\text{Area (sample)}}{\text{Wt \% standard}}$$

Precautions

1. Degas the solvent before use to remove dissolved gasses.
2. Use water HPLC grade.

Reference

Citrus Fruits and their Production: Analysis and Technology, By S.V. Ting and Russell L. Rouseff (1986). Marcel Dekker Inc. New York, pp. 88-90.

20

Organic Acid Determination by HPLC

Equipment and Operating Condition

An isocratic HPLC system consist of pump, C-18 column, detector and recorder its required. Either a refractive index detector or a UV detector set at 214nm may be used, Run time is 18 min. at a flowering of 0.5 ml./min.

Reagents

1.00 per cent citric acid standard is prepared by dissolving 1.53g of ACS reagent grade, Sodium citrate dehydrate in 100ml water. A separate 1 per cent of ACS grade I-malic acid is prepared in a similar manner. (This acid is available in a non-hydrated form). Mobile phase consist of 2 per cent potassium dihydrogen phosphate adjusted to pH 2.4 with phosphoric acid.

Sample Preparation

Centrifuge juice to remove pump and some suspended solution and dilute 1:10 with distilled water. Pre-condition a C-18 mini cartridge (Water sep pack of Baker 10 SPE 6ml column) with approximately 5 ml of methanol

(MeOH) followed by water (HPLC grade). Pass 4-5 ml of dilute centrifuged juice is passed through column and discarded. Slowly pass 2-3ml more of the same through the column and collect this portion, if final portion is not clear, it should be filtered through at 2μ filter, injection volume is 0.5μl.

Calculation

Prepare standard curve of peak height was acid concentration (wt per cent) for each acid. Determine the amount of acid present in a sample by measuring the peak height of each acid and determining its concentration from the respective standard curve.

Preacutions

1. Citric acid standard most be prepared accurately.
2. Juice should be cleanup before use in HPLC work.

Reference

Citrus Fruits and their Production: Analysis and Technology, By S.V. Ting and Russell L. Rouseff (1986). Marcel Dekker Inc. New York, pp. 92-93.

21

Determination of Thiabendazole in Fruit by UV Spectrophotometer

Reagents

1. Thiabendazole
2. Chloroform
3. Sodium hydrogen carbonate sodium 5 per cent m/v sodium bicarbonate
4. Hydrochloric acid 0.1 N
5. Sodium hydroxide solution
6. Trisodium citrate dihydrate
7. Sodium sulphate – anhydrous
8. pH indicator paper

   4 to 6

   8 to 10

   10 to 12

Preparation of Sample

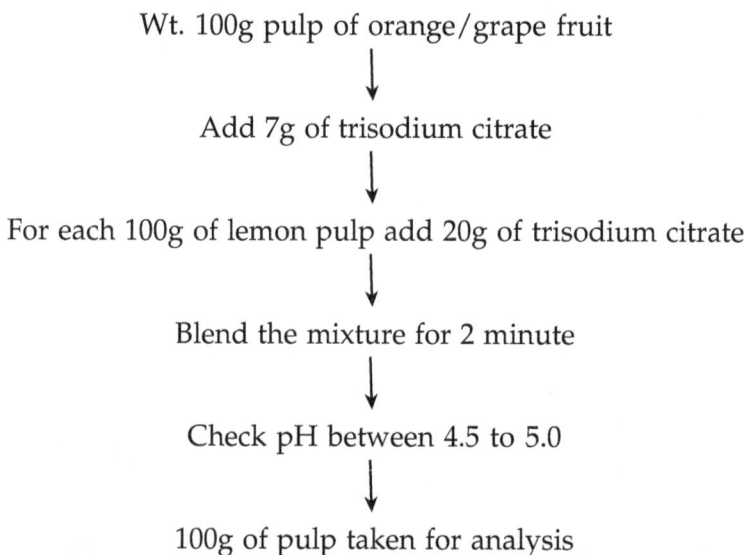

Wt. 100g pulp of orange/grape fruit

↓

Add 7g of trisodium citrate

↓

For each 100g of lemon pulp add 20g of trisodium citrate

↓

Blend the mixture for 2 minute

↓

Check pH between 4.5 to 5.0

↓

100g of pulp taken for analysis

Extraction of Thiabendazole

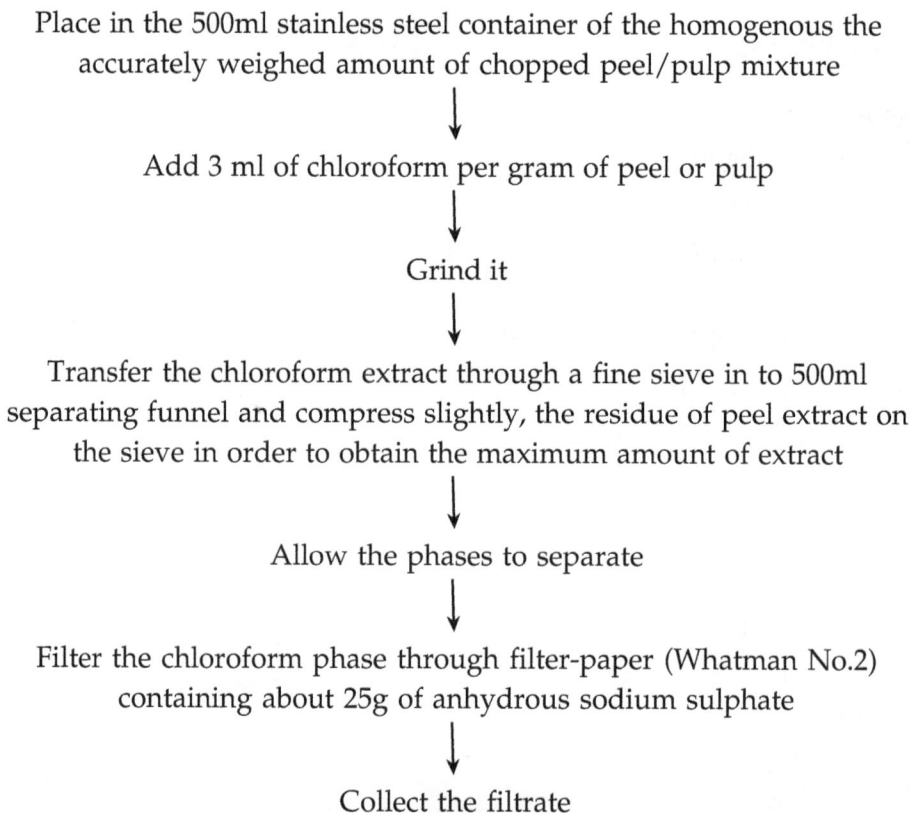

Place in the 500ml stainless steel container of the homogenous the accurately weighed amount of chopped peel/pulp mixture

↓

Add 3 ml of chloroform per gram of peel or pulp

↓

Grind it

↓

Transfer the chloroform extract through a fine sieve in to 500ml separating funnel and compress slightly, the residue of peel extract on the sieve in order to obtain the maximum amount of extract

↓

Allow the phases to separate

↓

Filter the chloroform phase through filter-paper (Whatman No.2) containing about 25g of anhydrous sodium sulphate

↓

Collect the filtrate

↓

Concentrate the extract at atompshpere pressure
to a volume of about 10-15 ml

Separation of Thiabendazole from the Bulk of Extractive Substances

Add to the extract 20ml of water and exactly 5ml of 0.1 N HCl

↓

and boil to eliminate completely the remaining chloroform

↓

Detach the flask from the conc. Apparatus and boil the
acidic mixture while exposed

↓

Concentrating it to approximately 10ml

↓

Cool and transfer the mixture quantitatively into a 25ml calibrated flask

↓

Rinsing the flask with D.W.

↓

Make the volume upto mark of 25 ml

↓

Mix the solution and filter carefully through a folded
Whatman filter paper No. 2

↓

The filtrate is almost colourless and should be sufficiently clear to avoid
the formation of an emulsion during subsequent extraction with
chloroform

Cleanup the Interfering Substances

Place exactly 20ml filtrate, which contains 4 ml of 0.1N HCl, into 100ml
separating funnel

↓

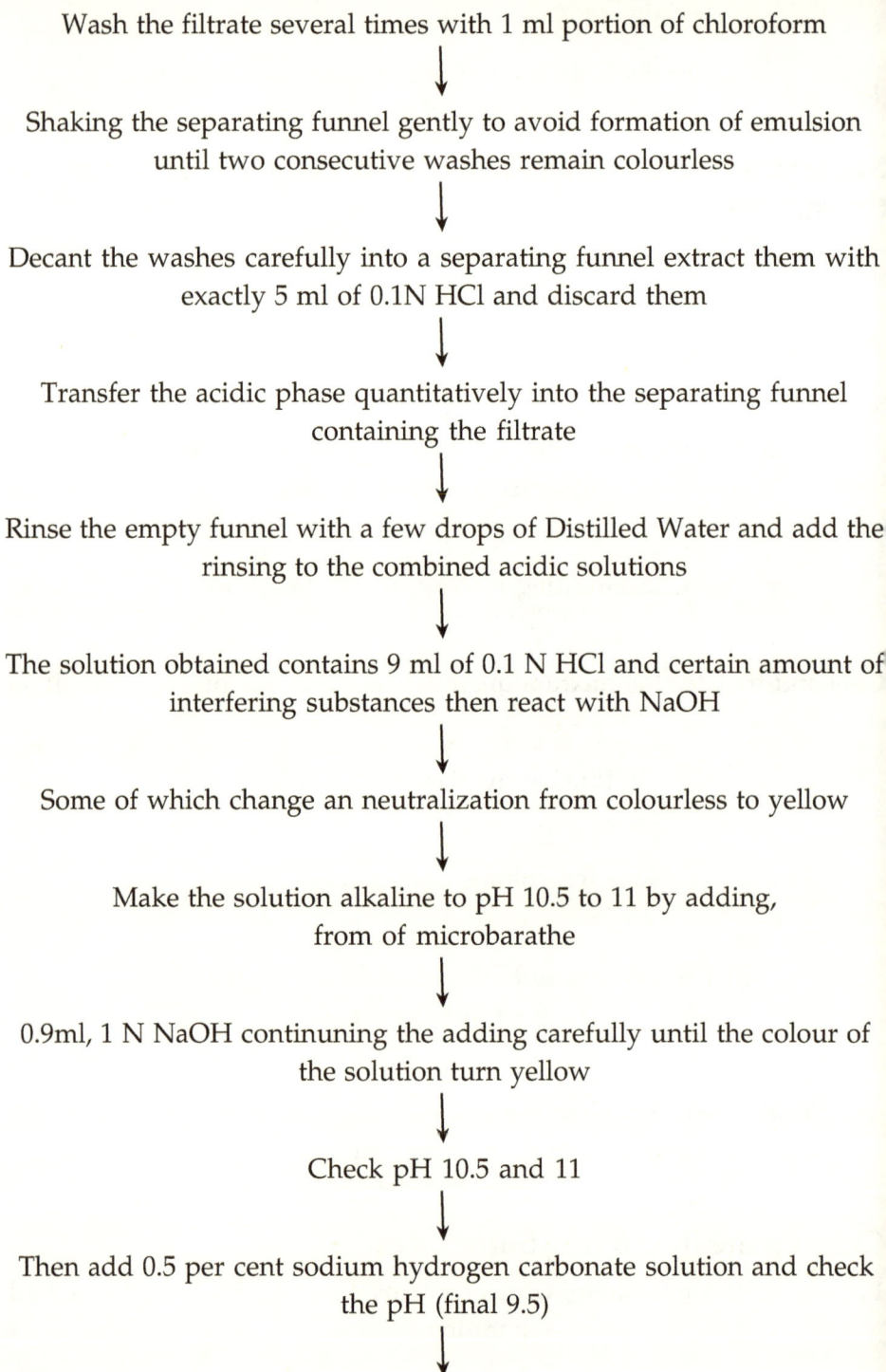

Wash the filtrate several times with 1 ml portion of chloroform

↓

Shaking the separating funnel gently to avoid formation of emulsion
until two consecutive washes remain colourless

↓

Decant the washes carefully into a separating funnel extract them with
exactly 5 ml of 0.1N HCl and discard them

↓

Transfer the acidic phase quantitatively into the separating funnel
containing the filtrate

↓

Rinse the empty funnel with a few drops of Distilled Water and add the
rinsing to the combined acidic solutions

↓

The solution obtained contains 9 ml of 0.1 N HCl and certain amount of
interfering substances then react with NaOH

↓

Some of which change an neutralization from colourless to yellow

↓

Make the solution alkaline to pH 10.5 to 11 by adding,
from of microbarathe

↓

0.9ml, 1 N NaOH continuning the adding carefully until the colour of
the solution turn yellow

↓

Check pH 10.5 and 11

↓

Then add 0.5 per cent sodium hydrogen carbonate solution and check
the pH (final 9.5)

↓

Extract the mixture 4 times with 5 ml portions of chloroform and decant the chloroform phases carefully into a 100ml separating funnel

↓

Discarding the aquous phase

↓

Extract the combined chloroform phase with extractly 1, 10 and 5 ml of 0.1N HCl

↓

After the first two extraction, decant the chloroform phase into a clean separating funnel and discard it after the third extraction and add quantitatively the second and third acidic extracts to be first extract, rinsing the empty funnel with a few drops of water

↓

Wash wth combined acidic extracts with three 1 ml portion of chloroform

↓

Collect the washes in a separating funnel and extract them with 5 ml of 0.1N HCl

↓

Discard the chloroform phase and quantitive transfer the acidic phase into funnel containing the combined acidic extracts

↓

With a micro burette add 3.0 ml of 1N NaOH sodium and pH check 10.5 to 11

↓

Then add 0.5ml of 5 per cent sodium hydrogen carbonate solution and check the pH of the mixture (9.5)

↓

Extract it with five and to 5 ml portion of chloroform, collect the chloroform phases in a 25ml calibrated flask and make the volume up to the mark

$$\downarrow$$

Finally add anhydrous sodium sulphate mix, allow the mixture to stand and determine of the thiabendazole contents of the chloroform extract

$$\downarrow$$

Record O.D. 255 and 330nm

Standard

20mg thiabendazole/100 ml chloroform 0.1 to 15μm ml^{-1}

Precautions

1. Cleanup the interfering substances must be removed carefully.

2. Normality of HCl check properly to obtain better result.

Reference

Analyst, Feb. 1974 Vol-99 *Anna Rajzman* pp-120-127.

22

Determination of Peroxidase Enzyme (Donor : H_2O_2 Oxidoreductase EC 1.11.17)

Principle

Peroxidase (POD) catalyses the dehydrogenation of large number of organic compounds such as phenols, aromatic amines, hydroquinones etc.

Guaiacol o-dianisidine dye is used as substrate for the assay of peroxidase.

POD

Guaiacol + H_2O_2 $\longrightarrow$ Oxidized guiacol + $2H_2O$

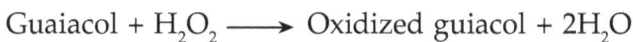

The resulting oxidized (dehydrogenated) guaiacol is probably more than one compound and depends on the reaction condition. The rate of formation of guaiacol dehydrogenation product is a measure of the POD activity and canbe assayed spectrophotometerically at 460 nm.

Reagents

1. H_2O_2 – 1 per cent
2. *O*-dianisidine dye 1 per cent in methnol
3. Potassium phosphate buffer 0.1M, pH 7.2 (chilled)

Procedure Extraction

0.5/1.0g sample grind in ice chilled mortar and pestle

$\downarrow$

Extract the enzyme with 0.1M phosphate buffer, pH 7.2 (chilled)

Substrate Mixture

Take 0.05 ml *O*-dianisidine dye in 6 ml 1 per cent H_2O_2

or

0.3 ml *O*-dianisidine dye in 36ml 1 per cent H_2O_2

Assay Reaction

Take 3ml of substrate + *O*-dianisidine dye in cuvette

$\downarrow$

Add immediately 1ml of enzyme extract

$\downarrow$

Shake well to start the reaction

$\downarrow$

Immediately kept the cuvette in vv-vis-spectrophotometer

$\downarrow$

Record the OD at 460 nm at every 10, 15 second to 180 second or until the solution of reaction turn brownish in colour

Calculation

Enzyme unit expressed as O.D. changes per minute

$$= \frac{60\,\text{Sec} \times \text{GF} \times \text{Total volume}}{\text{Aliquot taken (ml)} \times \text{Wt. of sample (g)} \times 1000}$$

Precautions

1. All extraction condition must maintain in ice-chilled condition.
2. If the rate of increases in very high, repeat the assay with dilute extract.

Reference

MC-Curne D.C. and Galstone, A.W. (1959). Invers effect of gibbelline on peroxidase activity during growth in dwarf strain of pea and corn. *Plant Physiology* 734 : 116-118.

23

Determination of Polyphenol Oxidase Enzyme (PPO) (Monophenol, Dihydroxy Phenylalanine Oxygen Oxidoreducaste EC 1.14.18.1)

Principle

Phenol oxidases are copper proteins of wide occurrence in nature which catalyse the acrobic oxidation of certain phenolic substrates to quinones which are autoxidized to dark brown pigments generally known as melanins, PPO comprises of catechol oxidase and lactose.

Reagent

1. Catechol – 110mg
2. Proline – 112 mg
3. Potassium phosphate buffer – 0.1 M, pH 6.5

Procedure

Extraction of Enzyme

Take 0.5 to 1.0g sample and ground it in pre chilled mortar and pestle

$\downarrow$

Extract the enzyme with 5 ml phosphate buffer 0.1 M pH 6.5 (chilled)

Substrate

Catechol – 110 mg

+

Proline – 112 mg   In 100ml phosphate buffer

+

Phosphate buffer 0.1 m pH 6.5

Enzyme Assay

Take 2.5ml of substrate in cuvette

$\downarrow$

Add 0.5ml of enzyme extract

$\downarrow$

Shake well, and kept the cuvette in spectrophotometer

$\downarrow$

Record the OD every 15 second interval till 180 seconds

Calculation

Enzyme unit is expressed as change in OD per minute

$$= \frac{GF \times 60\,Sec \times Total\ volume}{Enzyme\ aliquot\ taken \times Wt.\ of\ sample \times 1000}$$

Precautions

1. The enzyme concentration required to set satisfactory linearity of time vs absorbance decrease has to be standardized.

2. All condition must be maintain in ice-chilled condition.

Reference

Esterbauer, H. Schwagyl, F., Hayn, M. (1977). *Anal Chem.* 77 : 486.

24

Determination of Catalase Enzyme (Hydrogen Peroxide : Hydrogen Peroxide Oxidoreductase EC 1.11.1.6)

Principle

Catalase facilitates the dismutatio of H_2O_2 to water and O_2 according to the reaction.

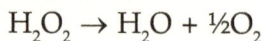

$$H_2O_2 \rightarrow H_2O + \tfrac{1}{2}O_2$$

The enzyme plays an important role in association with SOD as well as in photorespiration and glycolate pathwcy.

Reagent

1. Potassium phosphate buffer 0.1M pH 7.0
2. Potassium dichromate – acetic acid glacial (5 per cent potassium dichromate + alacial acetic acid in 1: 3 ratio)
3. H_2O_2, 0.2M (1.70 ml in 25ml Volume with D.W.)

Enzyme Extraction Procedure

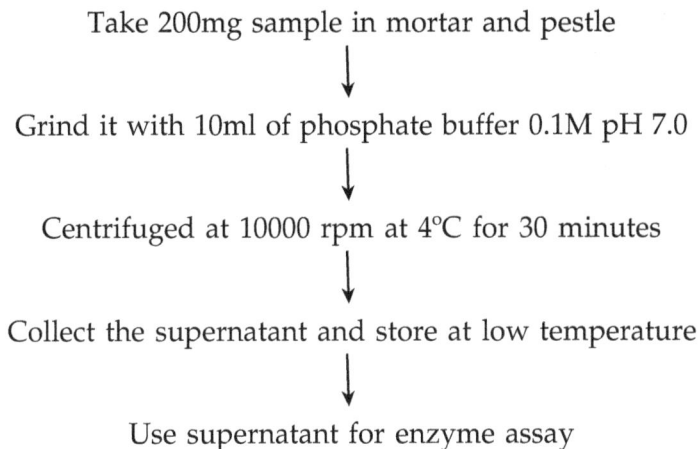

Take 200mg sample in mortar and pestle

↓

Grind it with 10ml of phosphate buffer 0.1M pH 7.0

↓

Centrifuged at 10000 rpm at 4°C for 30 minutes

↓

Collect the supernatant and store at low temperature

↓

Use supernatant for enzyme assay

Enzyme Assay

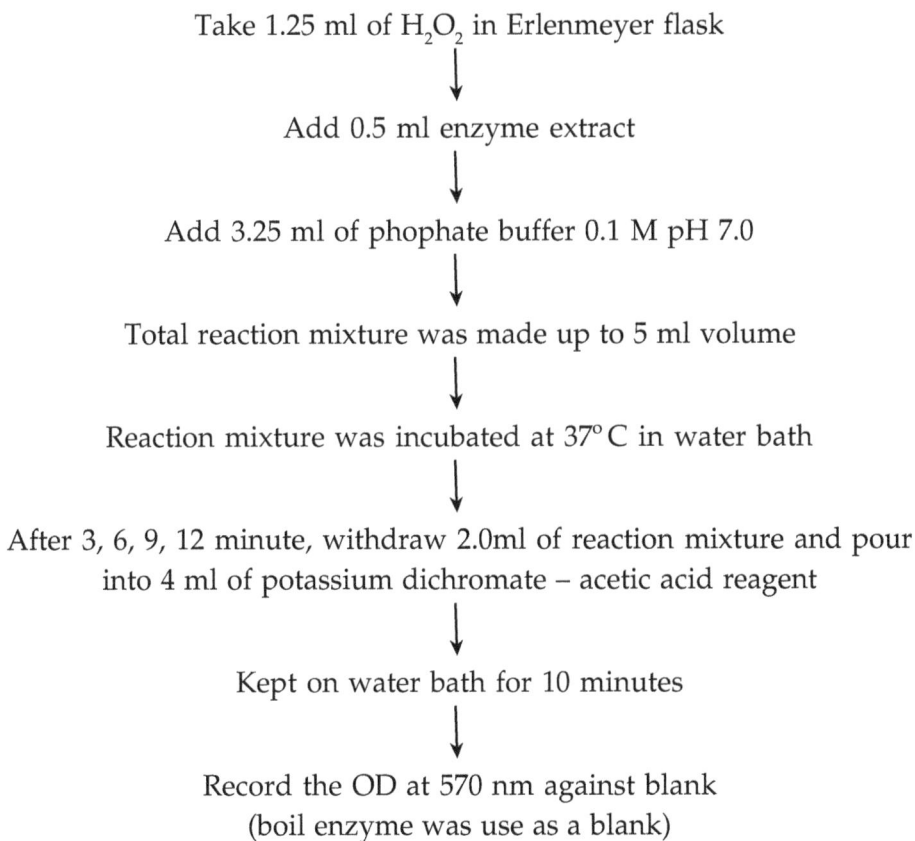

Take 1.25 ml of H_2O_2 in Erlenmeyer flask

↓

Add 0.5 ml enzyme extract

↓

Add 3.25 ml of phophate buffer 0.1 M pH 7.0

↓

Total reaction mixture was made up to 5 ml volume

↓

Reaction mixture was incubated at 37° C in water bath

↓

After 3, 6, 9, 12 minute, withdraw 2.0ml of reaction mixture and pour into 4 ml of potassium dichromate – acetic acid reagent

↓

Kept on water bath for 10 minutes

↓

Record the OD at 570 nm against blank
(boil enzyme was use as a blank)

The result were expressed as enzyme unit per gram fresh weight. One unit of enzyme activity is defined as amount of enzyme which produces an increase of OD per minute of incubation.

Precautions

1. Reaction mixture of enzyme assay maintain accurately 5 ml volume.

2. All assay condition must be maintain ice-chilled condition.

Reference

Kar, M. and Mishra, O. (1976). Catalase, peroxidase and polyphenol oxidase activity during rice leaf senescence *Pl. Physiol.* 57 : 315-319.

25

Isolation of Plant Genomic DNA by C-Tab Method

Principle

Agarose forms a gel by hydrogen binding and the gel pore size depends on the agarose concentration. The DNA molecules are seprated by electrophoresis on the basis of their size and the magnitude of net charge on the molecules. The dye ethidium bromide intercalates between the bases of RNA and DNA and fluorescence orange when irradiated with UV light. Low concentration agarose gels with large pore permit fractionation of high MW modecules and vice-versa.

One of the most widely followed extraction procedure involves the use of nonionic detergent cetyltrimethyl ammonium bromide (CTAB) which complexs with carbohydrates and can be phenol extracted. It is relatively simple procedure and is useful for the preparation of small samples of DNA needed for various applications such as PCR cloning etc.

Reagent

   a. Grinding buffer (for 100ml stock solution)

   CTAB – 3g

IM Tris – 10ml

EDTA – 4ml

5M NaCl – 28 ml

PVP – 2g

β-mercaptoethanol – 35 μl

b. Chloroform : isoamyl alcohol

Chloroform and isoamyl alcohol were mixed in ratio of 24:1.

c. TAE buffer (1xTAE per litre) pH 8.0

Tris base – 4.84g

0.5M EDTA pH 8.0– 2ml

Glacial acetic acid – 1.142ml

d. TE Buffer pH 8.0 (100 ml)

1 M Tris – 1 ml

0.5M EDTA – 200 ml

e. Loading dye (1x)

100 per cent glycerol – 0.7 ml

0.5M EDTA – 0.3 ml

Pinch of bromophenol blue was added in above 1 ml volume

f. Ethidium bromide

Ethidium bromide – 0.1g

Disttilled Water – 10ml

It was stored in dark bottle at room temperature

g. 0.5 M NaCl

h. Isopropanol

i. Liquid nitrogen (-196°C temp)

Procedure

50-100 mg fresh leaf/tissue sample were taken and grind in liquid N_2
with the help of morter and pestle

↓

Powdered leaves were taken in eppendrof tube

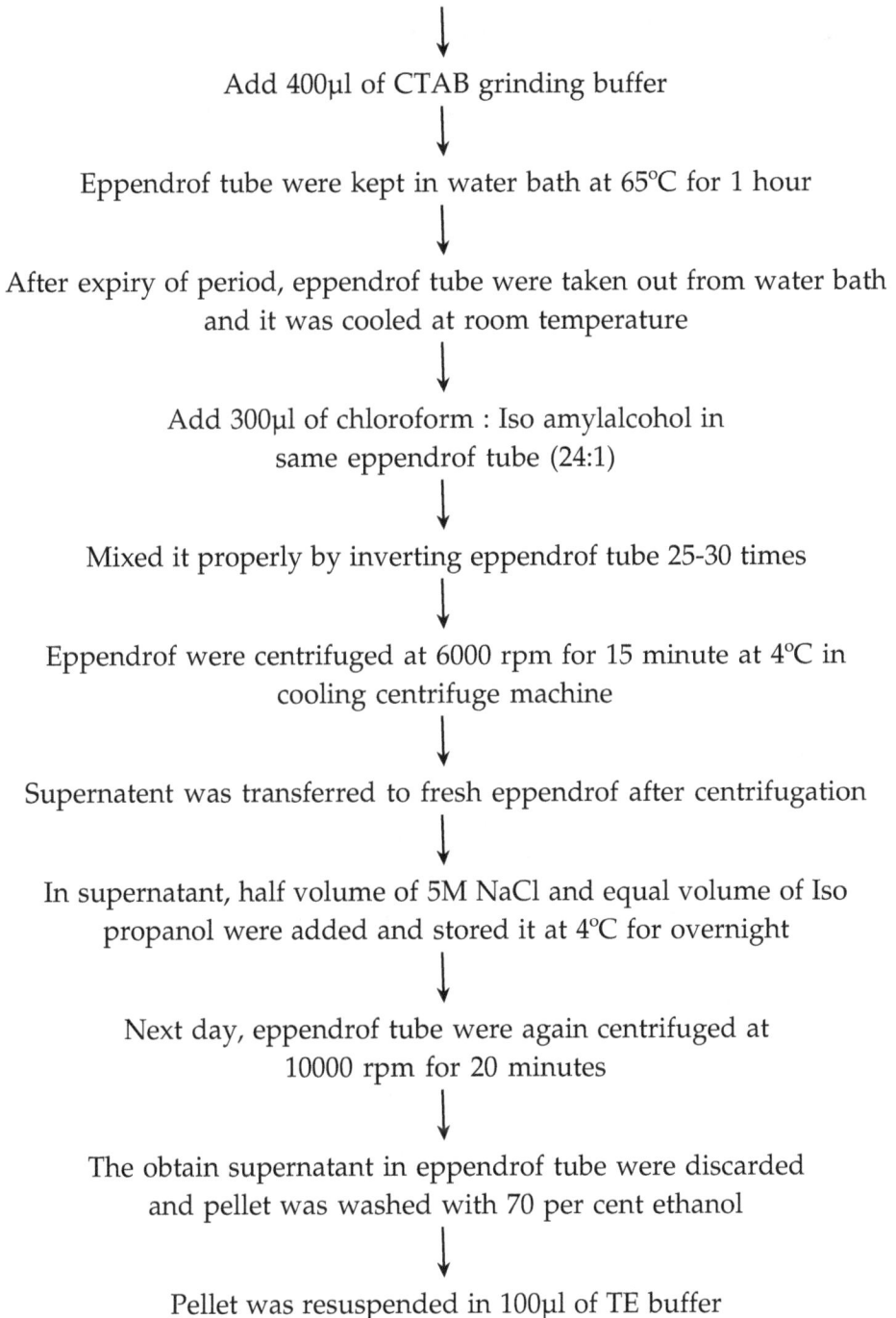

$\downarrow$

Add 400µl of CTAB grinding buffer

$\downarrow$

Eppendrof tube were kept in water bath at 65°C for 1 hour

$\downarrow$

After expiry of period, eppendrof tube were taken out from water bath and it was cooled at room temperature

$\downarrow$

Add 300µl of chloroform : Iso amylalcohol in same eppendrof tube (24:1)

$\downarrow$

Mixed it properly by inverting eppendrof tube 25-30 times

$\downarrow$

Eppendrof were centrifuged at 6000 rpm for 15 minute at 4°C in cooling centrifuge machine

$\downarrow$

Supernatent was transferred to fresh eppendrof after centrifugation

$\downarrow$

In supernatant, half volume of 5M NaCl and equal volume of Iso propanol were added and stored it at 4°C for overnight

$\downarrow$

Next day, eppendrof tube were again centrifuged at 10000 rpm for 20 minutes

$\downarrow$

The obtain supernatant in eppendrof tube were discarded and pellet was washed with 70 per cent ethanol

$\downarrow$

Pellet was resuspended in 100µl of TE buffer

Preparation of Gel for Electrophoresis

Isolated DNA were checked by agarose gel electrophoresis, for this purpose 0.8 per cent agarose gel was casted

↓

0.8g agarose was dissolved in 100ml TAE (IX) buffer and heated in micro oven

↓

Pinch of ethidium bromide (0.01 g/ml) was added in mild heated agarose solution

↓

Gel casting tray was put on plain surface comb was set at right position and finally melted agarose was poured in casting tray

↓

It was allowed to polymerase for 45 minutes

↓

After solidifying the get, comb was removed and tray placed in buffer tank in IX TAE buffer

Loading of Sample in the Wells

10 μl DNA sample mixed with 10 μl loading dye, mixed properly and loaded in well with the help of micro pipette

↓

After proper loading, electrophoresis unit was connected with power pack at 40mA for three hours

Gel Analysis

Gel was finally visualized on gel documentation system and band appear in gel is compared with standard band and expressed as base pair (bP).

Purity Test of DNA

In a spectrophotometer, check the optical density (OD) of a dilution of the DNA preparation at 260 and 280 nm. Pure DNA has cn A_{260}/A_{280} ratio of 1.8-2.0 in 10nM Tris-HCl, pH 8.5. Strong absorbance at 280nm,

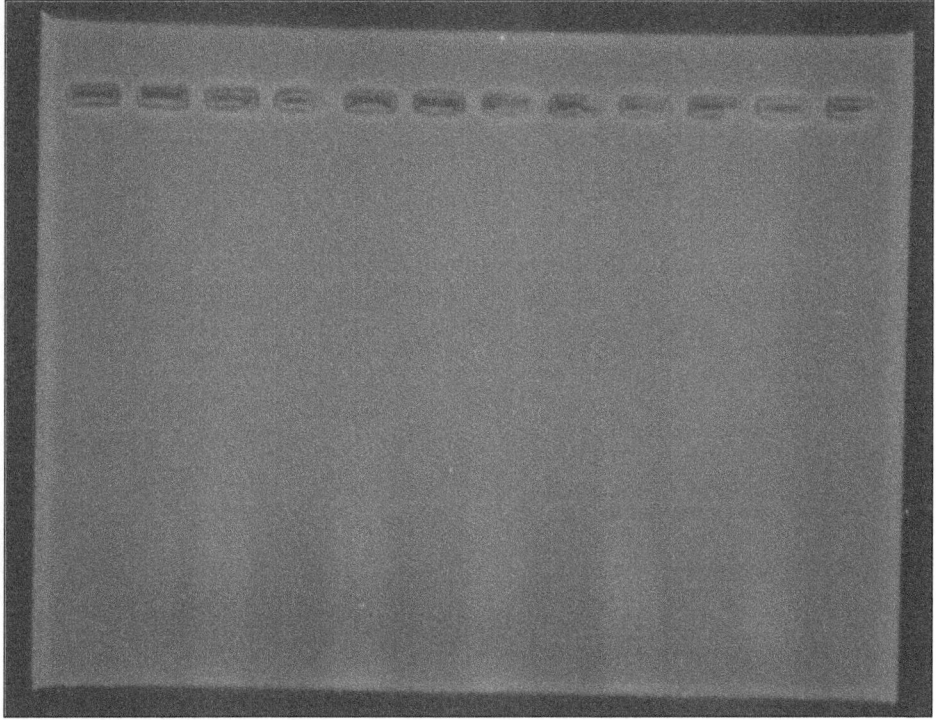

DNA/RNA on Agarose Gel Electrophorsis

resulting in a low A_{260}/A_{280} ratio, indicates the presence of contaminants such as proteins.

Conversion factor 50 to convert OD to concentration in µg/ml as DNA at a conc. of 50 µg/ml has a absorbance of 1 at 260 nm.

Precautions

1. Use fresh tissue to avoid DNA degradation due to old tissue, senescence.
2. Powder leaves in liquid N_2 do not contain moisture.
3. Ethidium bromide is a carcinogenic agent, so avoid direct contact with hand.
4. All the chemical glassware must be autoclave before DNA isolation.

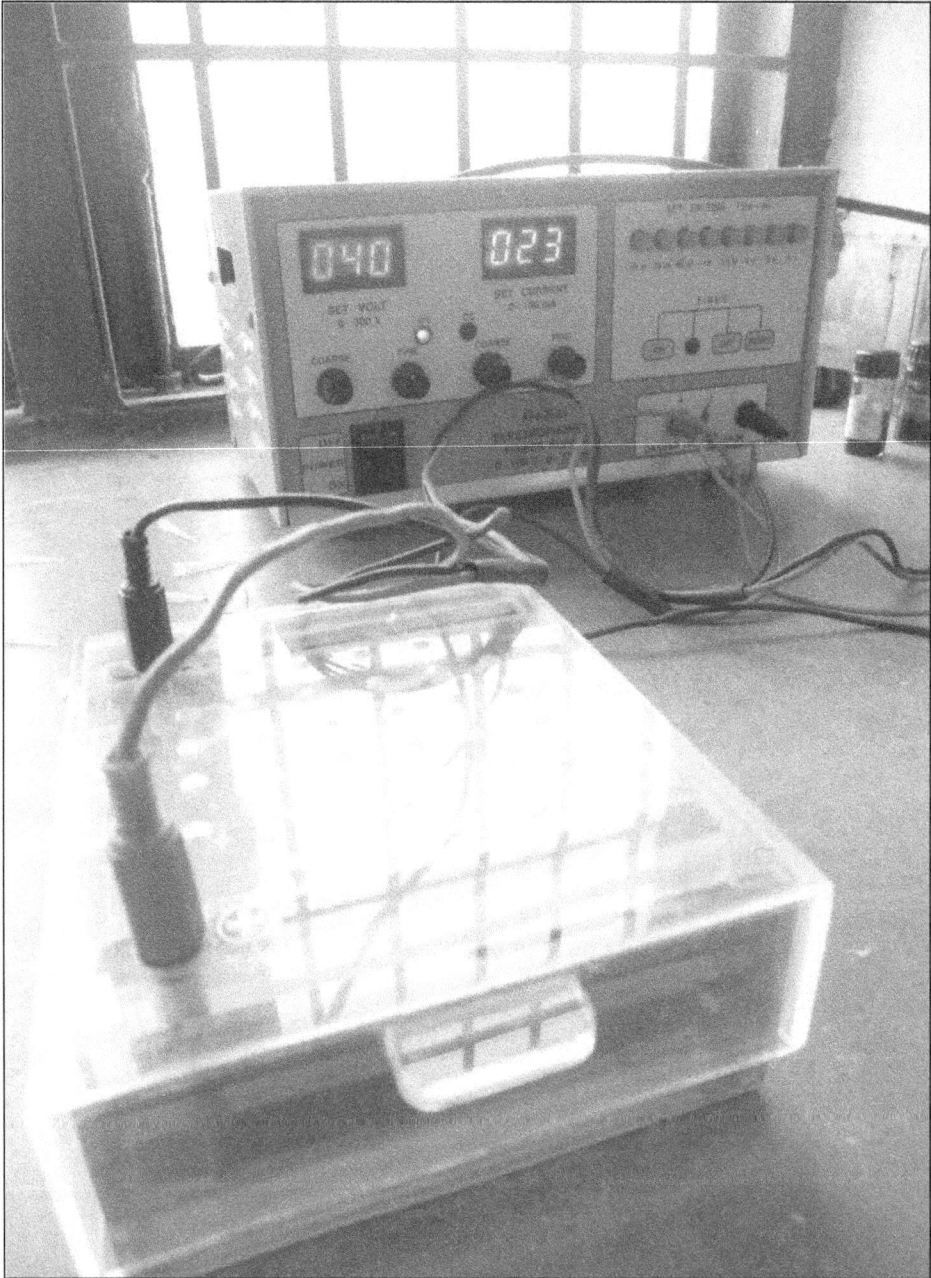

DNA Horizontal Gel Electrophoresis Unit

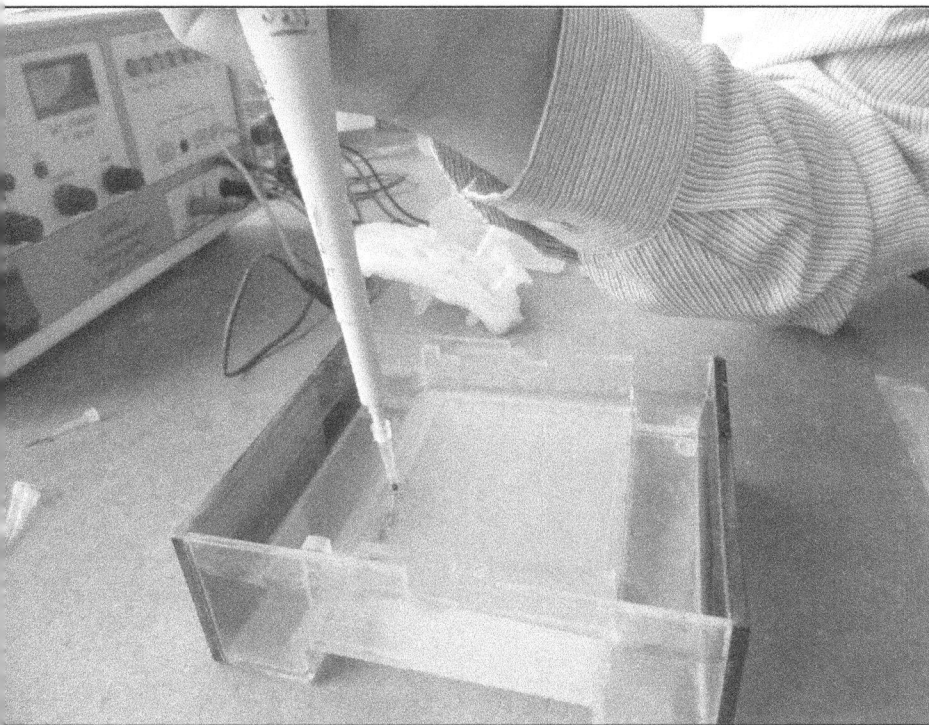

DNA Loading on Agarose Horizontal Gel Electrophoresis

References

Murray, M.G. and Thompson, W.F. (1980). Rapid isolation of high molecular weight plant DNA. *Nucl. Acids Res.* 8 : 4321.

Book: Sambrook, J., Fritsch, E.F. and Maniatis, T. (1989). *Molecular Cloning: A Laboratory Manual*, Cold Spring Harbor Laboratory Press, 3 Volumes.

26

SDS-PAGE Electrophoresis of Protein

Principle

SDS is an anionic detergent which binds strongly to and denatures protein. The number of SDS molecules bound to a polypeltide chain is approximately half the number of amino acid residues in that chain. The protein SDS complex carries net negative charge, hence more toward the anode when electrophoresed and the separations based on the size of the protein.

Apparatus

    a. Vertical slab gel type electrophoresis unit (Glass plate 18x9x0.1 cm) including power pack.

    b. Micropipette (10 – 1000 μl)

    c. Plastic tray for staining and destaining of gel

Reagent

    a. Stock Acrylamide Solution

       Acrylamide 30 per cent - 30g

Bis acrylamide 0.8 per cent - 0.8g

Distilled water – 100ml

b. Separating gel buffer

1.875M Tris – HCl – 22.7g pH 8.8

Distilled water – 100 ml

c. Stacking gel buffer

0.6M Tris HCl-7.26g pH 6.8

Distilled water – 100 ml

d. Polymerising agent

Ammonium per sulphate 10 per cent (100mg in 1 ml of distilled water)

TEMED (Fresh store in refrigerator)

(N, N, N, N, - Tetra methyl ethylene diamine)

e. Electrode buffer

0.025M Tris – buffer – 3.0g

0.192M glycine – 14.5g

0.1 per cent SDS – 1.0g

Made of with distilled water to 1000ml, adjust pH 8.2

f. Sample extraction buffer

0.1M Tris buffer – 1.21g/100ml Distilled water, pH 6.7

g. Bromophenol blue

0.5 per cent W/V solution in distilled water

diluted 1-5 times prior to use

h. Protein stain solution

Coomassie brilliant blue R-250 (CBB R-250) 0.25g in 80ml methnol, 20ml Acetic acid. To this was added 100ml distilled water (prepared fresh before use)

i. Destaining solution

7 per cent Acetic acid glacial

50ml methnol, add distilled water up to 100ml volume

Preparation of Gels for SDS – PAGE

a. Composition of Separating Get Buffer 10 per cent (30ml total volume)

1. Stock acrylamide – 10ml
2. Tris buffer 1.875M, pH 8.8 – 6.0 ml
3. Distilled water – 13.4 ml
4. SDS 10 per cent - 0.4 ml
5. Ammonium per sulphate – 150 µl
6. TEMED - 50 µl

Above solution was taken in flask and skaken well and contents transferred quickly into the chamber between the glass plates. The gel was left alone for polymerization (20-30 minutes).

b. Composition of Stacking Gel (Upper gel) 4 per cent Total Volume 10 ml

Stacking gel (upper gel) was prepared by mixing of the following solutions.

1. Stock acrylamide – 1.3ml
2. Tris buffer 0.6M pH 6.8 – 2.5 ml
3. Distilled water – 6.0 ml
4. SDS 10 per cent - 0.1 ml
5. Ammonium per sulphate – 100 µl
6. TEMED – 50 µl

Above solution was taken in flask and shaken well the solution was poured in the chamber containing polymerized running gel

↓

The comb was placed in between the plate and after complete polymerization of stacking gel in plate the comb was removed without distorting the shape of the well

↓

The glass plate with gel was assembled in electrophoresis unit containing electrode buffer in lower and upper tank of unit

Preparation of Sample

2g of tissue (sample) grind in 2ml of 0.1M Tris buffer pH 6.7 with the help of mortar and pestle

↓

Ground sample was transferred into centrifuge tube of 15 ml capacity

↓

Centrifuged at 5000 rpm for 10 minutes at 4°C

↓

After centrifugation, the supernetent (upper layer) was transfer into another centrifuge tube

↓

To this 0.2ml, 10 per cent SDS and 20µl merapto-ethenol were added

↓

Boil the sample on water bath for 2 minutes (ensure complete interaction between protein and SDS)

↓

After allowing to cool, 0.1ml of bromophenol blue dye and glycerol 1ml was added and mix it

↓

This sample was used for electrophoresis

Loading of Sample in to Well

40-60 µl of sample (containing about 75-200µl protein) was loaded into wells with the help of micropipettes

↓

Formation of bubbles was avoided during loading of samples

↓

After proper loading the electrophoresis unit was connected with power supply

↓

The current was trunned on allowing 30mA 220 volt for initial 10 minutes, until the sample travels through the stacking gel

↓

Then current was decreased upto 20mA till separation of proteins by electrophoresis

↓

After complete separation of protein when tracking dye reached the end of running gel, power supply was turned off

↓

The gel was gently removed from the space between the plates and immersed in staining solution contained in a plastic tray

Staining and Destaining of Gel

Gel immersed in staining solution (CBB R-250) contained in a tray, the tray was periodically shaken for uniform staining and this was continued for at least 1 hour

↓

The gel was destained by putting it in 7 per cent acetic acid and methanol solution

↓

Dye not bound to protein was removed

↓

The process was continued until background of gel become colourless

↓

The relative mobility of the different protein bands were recorded manually, or

↓

The bands was match with standard and protein markers (KD) loaded along the sample in gel

Precautions

1. Bubble should be avoid during preparation of gel.
2. As acrylamide is neurotoxic chemical it should not be touch by naked hand.

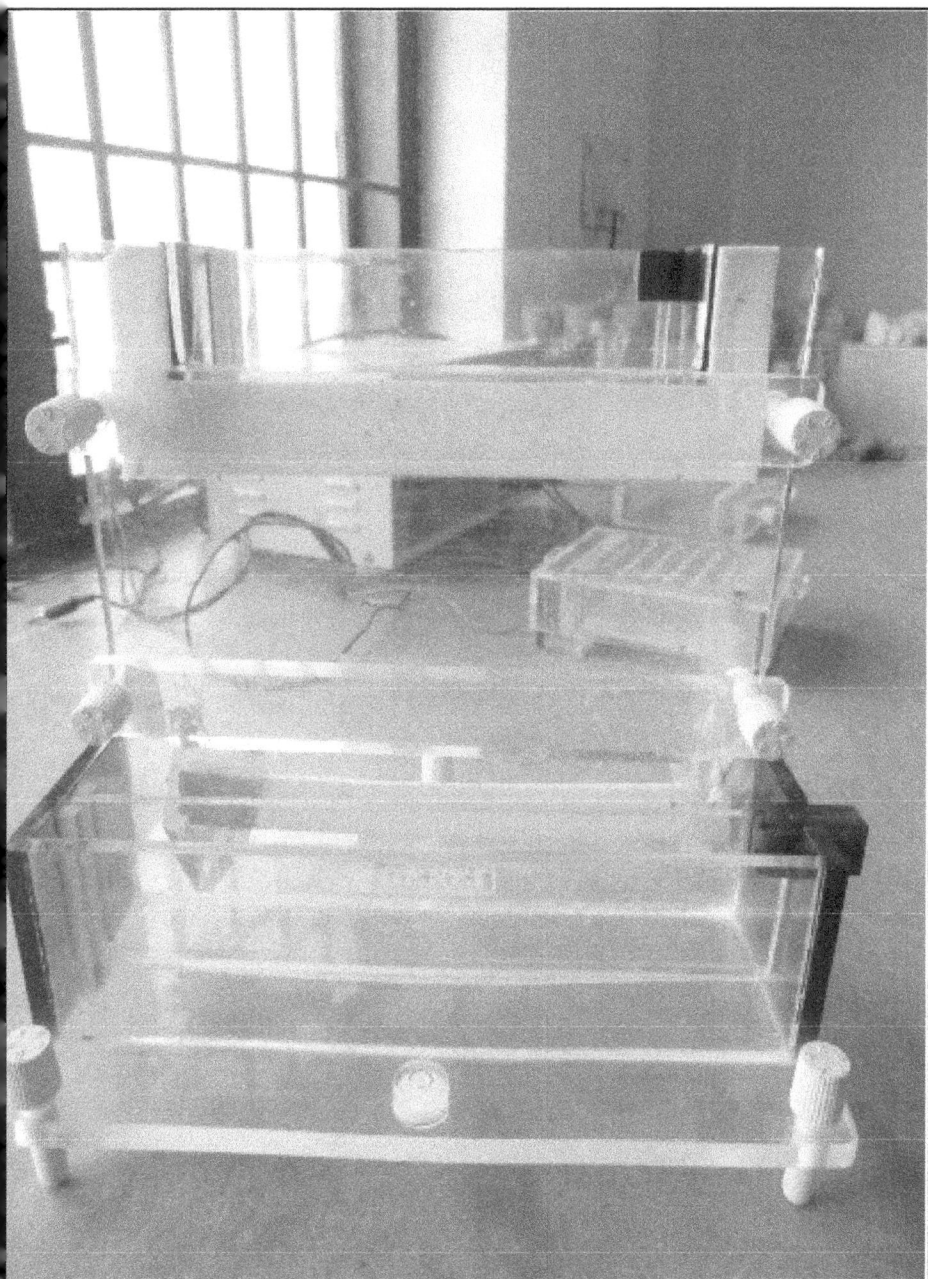

Vertical Slab Gel Electrophoresis Unit

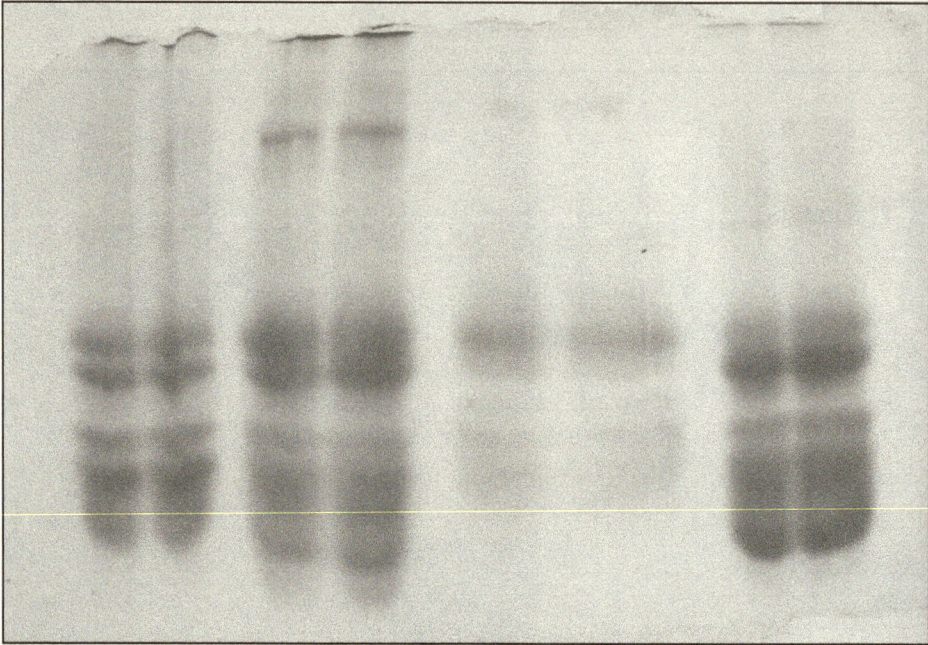

Protein Band in SDS-PAGE Electrophoresis

3. While deassmbling gel between glass plate, precaution should be taken to avoid breaking of gel.

4. Don't use excess persulphate to avoid wavy protein bands.

5. Protein concentration should not be below 0.1 µg protein.

6. Ammonium per sulphate should be prepared freshly.

7. TEMED must be kept air tight in refrigeration after use.

Reference

Laemmili, V.K. (1970), *Nature* 227 pp. 680.

Annexure-I

Definitions

1. **Atomic weight:** Atomic weight of an element is the relative weight of the atom on the basis of oxygen as 16.

   e.g.: Atomic weight of sodium is 23.

2. **Molecular weight:** The sum of the atomic weights of all the atomas in a molecule is its molecular weight.

   e.g.: Molecular weight of H_2SO_4 is 98, since

Hydrogen	2 x 1	=	2
Sulphur	1 x 32	=	32
Oxygen	4 x 16	=	64
			98

3. **Equivalent weight:** Equivalent weigh of a substance is the number of grams of the substance required to react with, replace or furnish one mole of H_2O^+ or OH $^-$.

   The equivalent weight of an acid is the weight that contains one atomic weight of acidic hydrogen *i.e.,* the hydrogen that reacts during neutralisatio of acid with base.

For example, the equivalent weight of H_2SO_4 is 49. Since H_2SO_4 contains two replaceable hydrogens, equivalent weigh of molecular weight/2 *i.e.*, 98/2 = 49.

4. **Percent solution (W/V):** One per cent solution of substance contains one gram of the substance in 100mL of the solvent. If v/v is given, it means 1 mL in 100 mL of solvent.

5. **Molar solution (M):** One molar solution of substance contains one mole or one gram molecular weight of the substance in one litre of solution.

   e.g. : 1 M NaOH contains 40g sodium hydroxide in one litre solution.

   Likewise, one millimolar solution of a substance contains one milligram molecular weigh of the substance in one litre of solution.

   e.g. : 1mM NaOH contains 40mg sodium hydroxide in one litre solution.

6. **Normal Solution (N):** One normal solution of a substance contains one equivalent or one gram equivalent weight of the substance in one litre of solution (*i.e.*, moleucar weight divided by the hydrogen equivalent of the substance).

   e.g.: 1 N H_2SO_4 contains 49g H_2SO_4 in one litre solution.

7. **Buffer:** A solution containing both a week acid and its conjugate weak base whose pH changes only slightly on the addition of acid of alkali.

8. **pH:** pH is a value taken to represent the acidity or alkalinity of an aqueous solution. It is defined as logarithm of the reciprocal of the hydrogen ion concentration of the solution.

   i.e. $\text{pH} = \log \dfrac{1}{[H^+]}$

9. **Dilute Acids:** While preparing dilute acids, add acid slowly to water preferably under cooling.

   Alkali Solution: When preparing concentrated alkali solutions (*e.g.*, 40 per cent NaOH) dissolve the alkali in distilled water under cooling.

10. **Water:** In biochemical experiments, it is advised to use distilled water for all purpose. So, water means distilled water in the methodologies given.

Concentration of Solution

Molarity (M)	:	The number of moles of solute per litre of solution (The term molar is equivalent to mol 1^{-1})
Molality (M)	:	The number of moles of solute per kg of solvent
per cent (w/v)	:	The weight in grams of solute per 100mL of solution
per cent (w/w)	:	The weight in grams of solute per 100g of solution

Unit of Length

1 micron = 1μ = $1\mu m$ = $1\times 10^{-6}m$ = $1 \times 10^3 nm$ = 1×10^4 Å

1 Å = 0.1nm = 1×10^{-4} μm = $1\ 10^{-10}m$

1nm = 10Å = $1 \times 10^{-3}\mu m$ = $1 \times 10^{-9}m$

Convert Units of Temperature

Temp. in °F = (Temp. in °C × 1.8) + 32

Temp. in °C = (Temp. in °F – 32) × 5/9

Temp. in K = (Temp. in °F + 459.67) × 5/9

Units of Radioactivity

Curie (Ci) =	that quantity of a radioactive substance in which 3.7×10^{10} atoms disintegrate in per second. Thus 1 Ci = 3.7×10^{10} dps= 2.22×10^{12}dps
Becquerel (Bq) =	That quantity of radioactive substance in which one atom disintegrates per secondThat 1Ci = 3.7×10^{10} Bq1Bq = 1 dps = 60 dpm

Some Isotopes and their Properties

Isotope	Type of Decay	Half-life	Average Energy
^3H	β^-	12.3y	0.0055
^{14}C	β^-	5570y	0.05
^{32}P	β^-	14.5d	0.70
^{35}S	β^-	87.4d	0.049
^{36}CI	β^-	3.07×10^5y	0.30

y: year; d: day.

Annexure-II

How to Prepare Reagent

1. How to Check Normality of Solution

a) How to Calculate Normality of HCl (12N)

HCl purity = 35.4 per cent

Mol. Wt. = 36.5

Specific gravity or density = 1.18

Mass = Volume × Density

= 1000 × 1.18 = 1180g = 1 L

$$= 1180 \times \frac{35.4}{100} = \frac{417.72}{36.5} = 11.4 = \sim 12 \text{ N}$$

b). How to Calculate Normality of H_2SO_4 (36 N)

Specific gravity = 1.84

Purity = 98 per cent

Eq. Wt. = 49

Mass = Vol. x density

= 1000 x 1.84 = 1840

$= 1840 = 1$ Lt.

$= 1840 \times \dfrac{98}{100} = \dfrac{1803.2}{49} = 36.8$ or ~36 N

2. ppm (mg/L)

$= \dfrac{\text{Desired ppm} \times \text{Desired volume}}{\text{Stock solution}}$

$e.g. \quad \dfrac{100\,\text{ppm} \times 500\,\text{ml}}{1000\,\text{ppm}}$

$= 50\text{ml}/500$ ml

ppm to per cent

$= \dfrac{\text{ppm value}}{10000} = \text{per cent}$

$\text{ppm to meq/L} = \dfrac{\text{ppm value}}{\text{Mol wt.}}$

3. Normal Solution

a) *e.g.* 2 N HCl=174.8 ml/L, 1 N HCl = 87.379ml HCl/L, 6N HCl = 524.27ml/L

$2\,\text{NHCl} = \dfrac{\text{Equivalent wt.} \times \text{Normality} \times 100}{\text{Sp. gravity} \times \text{Purity}} = \dfrac{36.5 \times 2 \times 100}{1.18 \times 35.4}$

$= 174.8\text{ml/L}$

b) $0.1\ \text{N}\ H_2SO_4 = \dfrac{49 \times 0.1 \times 100}{1.84 \times 98} = 2.71\text{ml}\ H_2SO_4/\text{L}$

c) Per cent solution = $CaCl \rightarrow 250\text{ml} \rightarrow 0.25$ per cent

$= \dfrac{0.25 \times 250}{100} = 0.0625\text{g}/250\text{ml}$

d) Molar solution *e.g.* NaOH 0.15N $\rightarrow$ 100ml

$= \dfrac{\text{Mol. wt.} \times M \times \text{Volume required}}{1000}$

$= \dfrac{40 \times 0.15 \times 100}{1000} = 0.6\text{g NaOH}/100\text{ml D.W.}$

4. Desired per cent Solution from stock solution

70 per cent PCA → 52 per cent PCA is required

$N_1V_1 = N_2V_2$

$70 \times V_1 = 52 \times 500$ ml

$V_{1=} = \dfrac{500 \times 52}{70}$

= 371.5 ml PCA is taken and vol. made 500 ml with D.W.

Annexure-III

SI Units of Mass

The SI unit of mass (weight) is given below

Weight	Symbol	Multiple of Gram	Lower Equivalent
megagram	M	10^6	1000 kilogram
kilogram	K	10^3	1000 gram
gram	g	1	1000 miligram
milligram			
	m		
		10^{-3}	
			1000 microgram
microgram	μ	10^{-6}	1000 nanogram
nanogram	n	10^{-9}	1000 picogram

Constants of Acids and Bases

Acid Base	Formula	Molecular Wt.	Commerical Concentrated Reagent		
			Specific Gravity	Per cent by Weight	Molarity (M)
Acetic acid	CH_3COOH	60.1	1.05	99.5	17.4
Ammonium hydroxide	NH_4OH	35.0	0.89	28	14.8
Formic acid	$HCOOH$	46.0	1.20	90	23.4
Hydrochloric acid	HCl	36.5	1.18	36	11.6
Nitric acid	HNO_3	63.0	1.42	71	16.0
Perchloric acid	$HClO_4$	100.5	1.67	70	11.6
Phosphoric acid	H_3PO_4	80.0	1.70	85	18.1
Sulphuric acid	H_2SO_4	98.1	1.84	96	18.0

Annexure-IV

Phosphate Buffer

Stock solution

A: 0.2 M solution of monobasic sodium phosphate (27.8g in 1000ml)

B: 0.2M solution of dibasic sodium phosphate (53.65g of Na_2HPO_4 x $7H_2O$ or 71.7g of Na_2HPO_4 x $12H_2O$ in 1000ml)

xmL of A, ymL of B, diluted to a total of 200ml

x	y	pH	x	y	pH
93.5	6.5	5.7	45.0	55.0	6.9
92.0	8.0	5.8	39.0	61.0	7.0
90.0	10.0	5.9	33.0	67.0	7.1
87.7	12.3	6.0	28.0	72.0	7.2
85.0	15.0	6.1	23.0	77.0	7.3
81.5	18.5	6.2	19.0	81.0	7.4
77.5	22.5	6.3	16.0	84.0	7.5
73.5	26.5	6.4	13.0	87.0	7.6
68.5	31.5	6.5	10.5	89.5	7.7
62.5	37.5	6.6	8.5	91.5	7.8
56.5	43.5	6.7	7.0	93.0	7.9
51.0	49.00	6.8	5.3	94.7	8.0

Annexure-V

Commonly Glass Wares Used in Practical

1. Volumetric flask – 25 – 1000 ml
2. Conical flask – 25 – 1000 ml
3. Measuring cylinder – 10 ml – 2000 ml
4. Reagent bottle (Autoclavable) – 50 – 1000 ml
5. Pipette (Glass) Blowout 0.1 – 10mlGraduated 0.1 – 10 ml
6. Test tube 10 – 15ml
7. Petridishes – (autoclavable)
8. Culture tube – 50ml
9. Vial – 10 – 20ml
10. Test tube stand
11. Micropipette a). 0.1 - 10µlb). 10-50 µlc). 50-1000 µl
12. Wash bottle – 250-1000 ml
13. Beaker – 50 – 2000 ml
14. Funnel
15. Surgical gloves

16. Plastic tray
17. Separatory funnel
18. Whatman No. – 1 filter paper

Annexure-VI

Commonly Instrument Used in Practical

1. UV – Visible spectrophotometer
2. Vertical slab gel electrophoresis
3. Horizontal gel electrophoresis
4. Gel documentation system
5. pH meter
6. Cooling centrifuge machine
7. Electronic balance
8. Hot air oven
9. BOD incubator
10. Micro oven
11. ELISA reader
12. Water bath
13. HPLC
14. GLC
15. Vortex mixture
16. Magnetic stirrer
17. Pasteur pipettes

Index